JONNY
BOWDEN'S
SHAPE UP
WORKBOOK

JONNY

EIGHT WEEKS TO

BOWDEN'S

DIET AND FITNESS SUCCESS

SHAPE UP

WITH RECIPES, TIPS, AND MORE

WORKBOOK

Jonny Bowden, M.A., C.N.S.

PERSEUS
PUBLISHING

Copyright 2002 © by Jonny Bowden
Library of Congress Catalog Card information is available from the Library of Congress.
ISBN: 0-7382-0515-X

Printed in the United States of America.
Perseus Publishing is a member of the Perseus Books Group

Text design by Jeffrey P. Williams
Set in 11-point Berkeley Book by Perseus Publishing Services

First printing, December 2001.
Visit us on the World Wide Web at http://www.perseusbooks.com

Perseus Publishing books are available at special discounts for bulk purchases in the U.S. by corporations, institutions, and other organizations. For more information, please contact the Special Markets Department at the Perseus Books Group, 11 Cambridge Center, Cambridge, MA 02142, or call (617) 252–5298.

Our deepest fear is not that we are inadequate.
Our deepest fear is that we are powerful and beyond measure.
It is our light, not our darkness, that most frightens us.
We ask ourselves, who am I to be so brilliant, gorgeous, talented, fabulous?
Actually, who are you not to be?

—NELSON MANDELLA

CONGRATULATIONS!

This workbook contains everything you need to start shedding fat *immediately* in the fastest and healthiest way possible.

The workbook contains all the *food lists, exercises,* and *assignments* that made the original Shape Up! program so successful. You don't need to read the previous book (*Shape Up! The Eight-Week Program to Transform Your Body, Your Health, and Your Life*) in order to begin this program (I'd love for you to read it, but it's not *necessary*). All you need to do is read the food lists on (page 45), start your to-do list, do the preassignments on (page 8), pick a start day, and begin.

Do the program exactly as directed and it will work for you.

I guarantee it.

When I first wrote *Shape Up! The Eight-Week Program to Transform Your Body, Your Health, and Your Life,* there was a lot of controversy and disagreement in the nutrition community about "low-carb" diets. But the conventional nutrition establishment is beginning to see the light. Many highly respected nutritional experts are now starting to publicly say that the USDA food pyramid—which is the basis of conventional nutrition advice—is a mess! What good is it to recommend six to eleven servings of grain if wheat makes you bloated? What good is recommending dairy if you don't tolerate the casein and lactose in most dairy products? And what good is continuing to recommend "low-fat" diets when they are clearly making an awful lot of people fatter than ever? Obviously, one size fits all does *not* apply to diets. (I'm not sure it applies to much else in life either, but it *definitely* doesn't apply to diets!) We need the ability to tailor-make diet and exercise plans to fit a wide variety of metabolic types, body types, biochemical makeups, and lifestyles.

And that's where the Shape-Up program comes in.

The Shape-Up program puts *you* in the driver's seat of your life. If you do these assignments exactly as written—even if you don't understand at first *why* you're doing them—I can guarantee you that you'll not only lose weight but you will come away with a deeper and more profound sense of your own power in the universe than you ever thought possible.

If you'd like to read more about this program, and understand some of the science and the theory that went into making it, by all means check out *Shape Up!* (Did I mention that I'd love for you to read it?) But if you're eager to get going and don't much care for all the nutritional theory and personal stories and motivational pep talks, you can just plunge right in and begin right here.

Let the games begin!

Warmly,
jonny

GETTING STARTED

Quick Start

1. Read "How to Use This Journal" (p. 4).
2. Read the food lists marked "A," "B," and "C" (p. 45). You'll be using them in your assignments. Remember that you do not have to make any drastic changes for now. Concentrate on the foods you're going to *add* to your diet on a regular basis.
3. Read and sign the contract (p. 7).
4. Start your personal to-do list. Just write down a couple of things you need to do this week (in the section labeled "To-Do List," p. 25).
5. Answer the questions in the Starting Assignments 1–6 (p. 8).
6. Choose a start date, call that Week One, Day One, and begin.

   On each day's page, fill in what you ate and what exercise you did. The first week you're only going to be walking, so you can read the rest of the section on exercise (p. 11) later on. Try to answer the "end-of-day" questions as often as possible

At Your Leisure

1. Read the full explanation of the exercise program. You will be adding one to two exercises a week. There are diagrams to explain how to do them.

   For advanced exercisers: You may use the suggested intermediate/ advanced routines laid out in the Exercise section (p. 21), or you may use your own routines.
2. Read the full description of foods and food lists (p. 45).
3. Read the explanation of the To-Do List (p. 25) so that you understand how to use it in your assignments.

4. Read the section on the self-evaluation questions (p. 31). For those who want to do even more with this aspect of the Shape-Up program (highly recommended but not necessary), I've included some of my favorite journaling exercises in the section called "Exercises: Not the Physical Kind" (p. 35).

How to Use This Journal

The journal is the key to this program.

It's your classroom and your teacher for the next eight weeks.

Wherever you are right now, that's the place to start. The journal can facilitate your progress whether you are an athlete or a complete beginner; whether you have ten pounds to lose or more than a hundred.

The journal is much more than a food diary, though obviously keeping records of what you eat is a big part of it. But the real value of the journal is to get you more in touch with your life—to make you more conscious and less reactive where food is concerned.

Let me explain.

It is impossible in the world we live in to lose weight and change your body by accident. It's a completely uphill battle, and it will not happen without *mindfulness* and *consciousness*. You're going to be making permanent lifestyle changes that affect not only your weight but your entire sense of well-being, and that's going to mean that you need to take a serious look not just at what you eat and how much you exercise but at the whole way you *think* and *feel* about those things. Just as breaking the grip of addiction isn't as simple as "just saying no," changing your body isn't as simple as telling yourself to "just eat less." (In fact, counterintuitive as it may be, eating *too* much less works directly *against* you in the war against fat!)

Changing your body takes you smack up against a mirror in which you are forced to confront a lot of areas in your life that many of us would just as soon not look at, let alone examine under a harsh light. But the truth is that if you don't *look* at those things, you are surrendering your power to *change* them. And if this program is about anything at all, it's about gaining that power back, not only over food but over all areas of your life.

This journal is a tool for letting you really see what's going on with you. Food is integrated into your life. So is exercise—or at least it *will* be by the time you're finished with the program. So how can you look at either of these areas—food and exercise—without also looking at the life they are a part of?

The answer is: You can't.

And that's what the journal is for.

At the beginning of each day, take a moment to answer the question at the top of the page: "What am I going to accomplish today?" Understand, we're not talking stuff like "bringing peace to the Middle East" here. Just take a moment to think about what you need to do today or what you'd like to get done. It can be anything from "do my workout" to "take the kids to soccer" to "close the Anderson deal" to "call my parents." The purpose of the exercise is to get you to develop the habit of *saying* what's going to happen and having it coincide with what actually *does* happen.

Because, make no mistake about it, *that* is the beginning of personal power.

At the end of each day, there are a few questions I'd like you to answer before going to bed. They're on a page called the "End-of-Day Questions." Let's be real: You're probably not going to answer these questions every single day of the eight weeks. Doesn't matter. Do the best you can. If you get to them each day, terrific. If not, do the exercise as often as you can. I've only left a short space for the answer to each question for a reason: I don't want this to be a big chore. Just reflect for a few seconds on each question, jot down what comes to mind, and move on. If for any reason on a given day one of these questions really sparks a "eureka" response and you need to say more, there's an extra sheet at the end called "anything more." Use it to complete whatever you can't fit on the "end-of-day" page. Remember, don't let this part of the day become an obstacle. The point is to increase awareness and consciousness, and for you to learn whatever lessons you need to learn to be in the moment, complete the experience, let go, and move on. The point is not to make you crazy or to give you more to do than you want or need.

Pick a start day for beginning the eight-week program. It doesn't have to be tomorrow. In fact, I'd prefer that you first take however much time you need to read over the section "Getting Started," fill out the contract, and answer the questions in the six short assignments on the following pages.

Get familiar with the format of the program and mentally prepare for the journey ahead.

Welcome to your new life. It's going to be your finest creation.

The Top Ten List of Things to Know About Shape Up

1. The more you participate, the more you get. Just like in life.
2. The more you give away, the more you benefit.
3. There are no stupid questions.
4. Everything is related. It's not all about weight or pounds. Even though you may think it is. Trust me.
5. Learn from every experience.
6. Most unhappiness with weight comes from the meaning you attach to it.
7. Accept what is in order to move on. *"What is, is. What ain't, ain't."*
8. Beating yourself up accomplishes nothing, except ruining your day.
9. Beauty, attractiveness, and sexuality come in all sizes.
10. Don't postpone joy.

THE CONTRACT

I want you to make this contract with yourself. It's an important part of this program. It's not a promise not to cheat, or to always "Think positive," or anything else like that. You're only promising one thing: to stay in the game. I'd like you to read it over carefully and fill it out and sign it. If you really want to go to the wall with this one, re-write it in your own hand. I want you to own it. Whatever it takes.

I, _____, promise to commit to this program by being willing to look honestly at my behavior and feelings, no matter what comes up, and to record them in my journal.

I, _____, promise that before I break any of the promises or ignore any of the assignments, I will sit down and re-read this contract.

I, _____, promise not to let toxic influences — including well-meaning friends — interfere with my resolve to complete this program.

I, _____, promise to remember the reasons I am doing this program in the first place, especially when I am tempted to stop doing it.

I, _____, promise to recognize the inevitable negative thinking and doubts that will certainly come up for me during the program and, while recognizing and honoring them as my feelings, will not empower them by allowing them to stop me. I will remember that "feelings are not facts."

I, _____, promise to keep my commitment to myself and will make my word law in the universe. I will not drop out without discussing this with at least one other person. I will not hide from what comes up for me and will find opportunity in everything that occurs, no matter how much I may feel like giving up.

Signed _____   Date _____

Starting Assignments 1–6

Starting Assignment 1

Make a list of three things you most like about your body.

(Hint: Don't say "nothing." That's not allowed. It can be anything from your skin to your fingernails to your smile to the shape of a particular body part. If you honestly can't think of one thing, make something up.)

1. _____
2. _____
3. _____

Starting Assignment 2

Make a list of three things you most dislike about your body (I know what you're thinking; no more than three!!).

1. _____
2. _____
3. _____

Starting Assignment 3

Make a list of three things you could do right now that would make a difference in your health or well-being today.

(Hint: These things could be as simple as refusing dessert just for tonight or cutting portions in half for just one meal. And here's a note to your "inner voice" that we talked so much about in the book *Shape Up!*: Don't invalidate whatever you come up with by saying, "Well, that wouldn't make that much of a difference." That's not what's important here. What's important here is that you list something—some tangible action—that would be a step, no matter how small, in the direction you want to go. We'll worry about how "big" or "important" it's going to turn out to be later.)

1. _____
2. _____
3. _____

Starting Assignment 4

Make a list of three things that you are giving up by not being fitter and having a body you can be happy in. What is it costing you?

1. _____
2. _____
3. _____

(If you're really ambitious and want some "extra credit," try tackling this one as well: What do you gain by keeping things the way they are? What's the hidden pay-off?)

Starting Assignment 5

What are five ways you could add activity to your life? If you're already active, what are five ways you could add *more* activity to your life?

(Hint: You don't have to do any of these yet. Just dream them up. Maybe it's as simple as walking one bus stop from your house. Maybe it's having an imaginary ten minutes a day to jump rope. If you can't think of any ways . . . keep thinking. Make something up. This is not an action plan, it's an exercise in visualization. Start writing!)

1. _____
2. _____

3. _____
4. _____
5. _____

Starting Assignment 6

Make a list of foods that you consider your downfall. Then ask yourself when they call to you the loudest. What are the biggest stressors that trigger unwanted eating for you? What foods do you reach for first? What situations (or people) trigger it? (Examples: M&M's and popcorn while watching TV; ice cream when I feel lonely; beer when I'm out with friends after work.)

Food	*Notes (People/Places/Things/Circumstances)*
1. _____	_____
2. _____	_____
3. _____	_____
4. _____	_____
5. _____	_____
6. _____	_____

EXERCISE

The Shape-Up program has two exercise components: walking and weight training. The first week you just walk. Beginning in the second week, you add on exercises from the weight training group until you get up to all seven exercises in the "circuit." Beginners should follow the exercise portion of the Shape-Up program just as it is written, but for intermediates or more experienced exercisers, I've included other options.

> Many people who begin this program have been exercising on their own for a while and may want to continue with their own exercise program at the same time they do the Shape-Up assignments (on food, keeping journals, self-evaluation questions, to-do lists). That's fine. I've also included some thirty-minute workouts that you might want to try. Feel free to experiment. The important point to remember is that this is a graded program in which each week builds on the week before, so you're always set up for a win. Don't choose to begin at a level of exercise intensity that you won't be able to sustain. In fact, many people who have been exercising hard find it useful to "drop back" a little for the first few weeks while they work on the other aspects of the program. You can always "up the ante" as you move forward during the eight weeks.

Note to intermediate and advanced exercisers: You may already be doing exercise that you feel is a lot harder than what's in the beginning weeks of this program. Here's the deal: You can continue with what you're doing (see above), but I'd like to suggest that you actually "cut back" and start with the easier program I will outline. Here's why: There's a lot of stuff to do in these eight weeks. You're going to be learning to integrate a number of things in your life—eating, exercise, reflection, relaxation, and self-examination. By the end of the program, you will have developed a lifestyle change that you can live with that pulls together a lot of different elements that relate to both your physical and mental health. If you turn down the intensity just a bit at the beginning, you will be better able to focus on all of the elements of the program instead of burning out on the exercise part. Less intensity will also lower your stress hormones, which can have a profound effect on your weight. Don't worry, it gets more difficult. By the end of the eight weeks you'll be working out just as hard as you're doing now, if not harder, but you'll be much more mindful of how everything works together to achieve the body and life that you want.

> When beginning an exercise program, set yourself up for a win. Understand that you are building a habit—doing *something* consistently is more important than *what* you do.

These are the exercises and routines that make up the exercise portion of your weekly assignments:

CRUNCHES

Lie on the floor with your legs bent, feet flat on the floor and hands clasped behind your head with the elbows touching the ground. Your head should be in position with the body so that you could hold an apple between your chest and your chin .

Imagine Velcroing your lower back to the floor. You may feel like you're doing a small pelvic thrust slightly forward to accomplish this. Keep your lower back nice and stable in this position.

Curl your upper body forward and up holding the highest position for a full second before lowering your upper body back to the ground.

Don't pull on your neck when you come up.

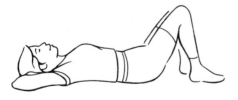
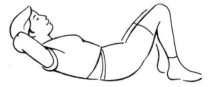

When you lower your upper torso back to the ground, don't return all the way to the "relaxed" position where your weight is supported by the ground, but rather to a point where your upper body is just above the ground and the abs are still contracted.

Remember to keep your elbows all the way back while doing the motion.

Repeat for as many reps as you can manage in good form. The goal is to try for 10–20 repetitions.

Note: I constantly hear from people that they are doing hundreds of crunches. The minute I hear this, I know they're doing them wrong. (I also know there's a good chance they're using momentum and are setting themselves up for a lower back injury.) If you do a crunch properly, it's hard. Most people don't do them correctly. The good news is that when you do them correctly, you don't have to do nearly as many to get results.

Beginners: Remember that if you can only do 1 or 2, that's fine. We'll work up to more, you can bet on it. Don't dwell on what you *can't* do, concentrate on what you *can* do.

SQUATS

Stand with your arms at your sides.

Keep your feet shoulder-width apart and your head up. There can be a slight arch in your lower back. Slowly bend your knees while pushing your rear out, until your thighs are about parallel to the ground. Squeeze your thighs and glutes for added contraction. At the same time as you bend, bring

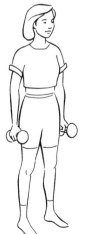
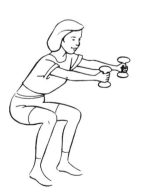

your arms up straight in front of you for balance till they're extended straight out at shoulder height, palms facing each other.

Now come up until you're standing again, dropping your arms back to your sides as you come up, and repeat for 10–15 reps.

Don't lock your knees when you return to standing position. Adjust your foot stance until it feels comfortable.

You're going to perform one set, from 8 to 15 repetitions. (Remember that if you can do only a few repetitions to start, that's fine too—that will be your personal starting point. You'll work up to where you can do 8–15.)

CHEST PRESSES

Lie down on a bench, your feet resting comfortably on the floor. (If you don't have a bench you can use a step or even the floor.)

Extend your arms overhead, shoulder-width apart, palms facing out, so that the dumbbells are positioned directly over your shoulders.

Bend your elbows about 90 degrees, gradually lowering the weights until they are above and a little beyond your shoulders.

Now push the dumbbells up with an arcing motion until they're back in starting position.

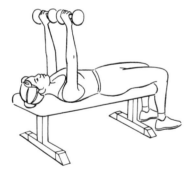 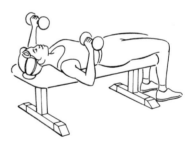

ONE-ARM ROWS

Bend over and rest your left hand on a bench or stool about 2.5-feet high. Extend your right leg behind you so that you're far enough away from the bench that your back is flat; make sure you don't round your back and instead keep it as flat as possible (you may actually have to arch it a little to keep it in this position). The right arm will be hanging down, straight. Your back should be like a table top in this position.

Take a dumbbell (or water bottle) in your right hand and bring it straight up toward your hip by bending your elbow and bringing it up behind you toward the ceiling. It should be almost like starting a lawnmower in slow motion. When the weight is about at hip level, lower it back down till the arm is hanging straight down. That's one "rep." After you complete the number of reps with your right arm, reverse everything and do the same number of reps with the left arm.

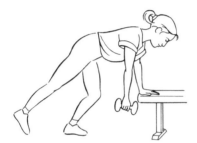 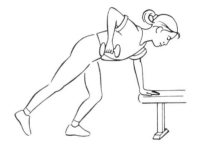

BICEP CURLS

Stand with a pair of dumbbells in your hands, palms facing out and feet shoulder-width apart.

Keeping your elbows stable, raise the dumbbells toward your shoulders and then bring them slowly back down. Repeat for 8 – 12 reps.

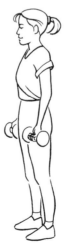 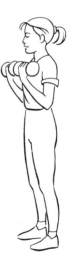

TRICEP DIPS

Sit on the edge of a bench or step, with your hands on the edge of the bench and fingers facing forward.

Lift your butt off the bench and lower it toward the floor by bending your arms at the elbows. Make sure you stay perpendicular to the ground, back straight. Don't push the hips forward.

Lift yourself back up by straightening your arms, but don't rest your butt back on the bench until you're done. Repeat for 8–12 reps.

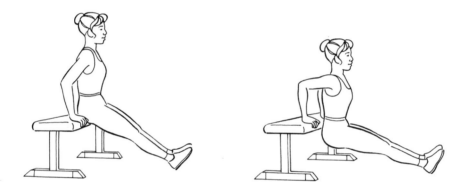

LATERAL RAISES

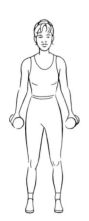
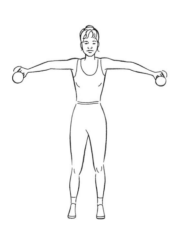

Take a dumbbell in each hand and hold at the sides of your body, palms facing inward. Stand with feet shoulder-width apart, knees slightly bent. Don't lean backward.

Raise your arms up and out to the sides till they are parallel to the ground, or "crucifix" position, then lower back down. Repeat for 8–12 reps.

(These are alternative workouts for advanced exercisers that can be substituted as noted in the exercise assignments beginning with week two. If you do the basic Shape Up! program as written or if you are a beginner, just stick with the exercise assignments as written and skip the options that follow for intermediate to advanced exercisers.)

WORKOUT "A"

Home Version	Gym Version
20 minutes of cardio	20 minutes of cardio
Squats (1 set)	Push-ups (1 set)
One-arm rows (1 set)	Squats (1 set)
Push-ups (1 set)	One-arm rows (1 set)
Leg presses (1 set)	Chest presses, regular or incline (1 set)
Lateral pull-downs (1 set)	Leg presses (1 set)
Chest presses, regular or incline (1 set)	Lateral pull-downs (1 set)
Crunches (2–3 sets)	Crunches (2–3 sets)
Stretch and cool-down	Stretch and cool-down

WORKOUT "B"

Home Version	Gym Version
20 minutes of cardio	20 minutes of cardio
Shoulder presses or lateral raises (1 set)	Shoulder presses or lateral raises (1 set)
Bicep curls (1 set)	Bicep curls (1 set)
Tricep dips (1 set)	Tricep push-downs (1 set)
Shoulder presses or lateral raises (1 set)	Shoulder presses or lateral raises (1 set)
Bicep curls (1 set)	Bicep curls (1 set)
Tricep dips (1 set)	Tricep push-downs (1 set)
Crunches (2–3 sets)	Crunches (2–3 sets)
Stretch and cool-down	Stretch and cool-down

WORKOUT "C"

Home Version	Gym Version
20 minutes of cardio	20 minutes of cardio
Shoulder presses or lateral raises (1 set)	Shoulder presses or lateral raises (1 set)
Bicep curls (1 set)	Bicep curls (1 set)
Tricep dips (1 set)	Tricep push-downs (1 set)
Shoulder presses or laterals raise (1 set)	Shoulder presses or lateral raises (1 set)
Bicep curls (1 set)	Bicep curls (1 set)
Tricep dips (1 set)	Tricep push-downs (1 set)
Crunches (2–3 sets)	Crunches (2–3 sets)
Stretch and cool-down	Stretch and cool-down

10-Minute Workouts

The biggest obstacle to the 10-minute workout lives in your mind. It's the idea that if you "only" do 10 minutes, it doesn't count. It does. Although it's true that you can get a lot of benefit out of longer workouts, it's equally true that 10 minutes "counts" and that it all adds up at the end of the day. If you've only got 10 minutes or so on a given day, here are four examples of what you can do effectively. The possibilities are limited only by your imagination.

Low-Intensity (at home, no equipment required)

1. March in place for 1–2 minutes.
2. Wall push-up: Stand about an arm's length away from a wall; extend both arms out and place both hands on the wall, shoulder width apart. Elbows are shoulder level. Now lean in toward the wall, bending the elbows as you come forward, and straightening the elbows as you push away, back to the starting position. Do 10 repetitions.

3. Squats to a chair: Stand approximately 8–12 inches away from a chair, facing away from the seat. Now bend your legs, push your butt out, and bend forward till you are seated on the chair. Beginners—rest for a second, then put your hands on your thighs, push off using your legs, and stand. Do 10 repetitions. Nonbeginners—just let your butt touch the seat of the chair and come right back up, keeping tension on the muscles throughout the movement.

4. Wall push-up (repeat, 1 set, 10 repetitions)

5. Squats to a chair (repeat, 1 set, 10 repetitions)

6. Free dance: This can be anything you want it to be. You can sway to soft music or you can pretend to be Brittney Spears. Think Tom Cruise in *Risky Business*. No one's watching. Have fun. Dance for 3 or 4 minutes.

7. Cool down, lie down, stretch, and breathe for 1 or 2 minutes.

High-Intensity (in home, equipment not needed)

1. Walk in place, light calisthenics: 1 minute
2. Jump rope: 2 minutes
3. Push-ups: all you can do in 1 minute
4. Crunches: all you can do in 1 minute
5. Jump rope: 2 minutes
6. Push-ups: all you can do in 1 minute
7. Crunches: all you can do in 1 minute
8. Relax and breathe: 1 minute

Moderate-Intensity Cardio Workout (outdoors or on a treadmill)

Hint: You can turn this into a high-intensity workout by picking up the pace on the running intervals, and you can lower it a bit by changing the running intervals into fast walks.

1. Walk for $1\frac{1}{2}$ minutes, gradually picking up pace
2. Run for thirty seconds
3. Walk for $1\frac{1}{2}$ minutes
4. Run for thirty seconds

5. Walk for 1½ minutes
6. Run for 30 seconds
7. Walk for 1½ minutes
8. Run for 30 seconds
9. Walk, gradually slowing down, for 2 minutes

The Moderate -ntensity Weight Training Workout (gym-based)

1. Light calisthenics, or 1 minute on stationary bike
2. Chest presses (1 set, 12–20 reps)
3. Seated rows (1 set, 12–20 reps)
4. Shoulder presses (1 set, 10–15 reps)
5. Bicep curls (1 set, 10–15 reps)
6. Tricep press-down (1 set, 10–15 reps)
7. Leg extension (1 set, 12–20 reps)
8. Hamstring curls (1 set, 12–20 reps)
9. Crunches, (1 set, 15–25 reps)
10. Relax and breathe (approx. 1–2 min)

The "No-Frills," "No-Excuse," Anytime, Anywhere Workout

This is my personal solution to the "time demon," my own "no-excuse" workout. I like it because it takes as little as 15 or 20 minutes, but it's easily expandable to 30 or 40, and it can be done by beginners or by advanced exercisers. It can be done anywhere—a gym with a treadmill is nice, but not necessary. A park or a city block in combination with four feet of floor space in a living room will do just as well. A little twiddling will let you customize this workout to virtually any time slot and fitness level.

Here 'tis:

1. Run a mile
2. Do some squats
3. Do some push-ups

4. Do some crunches

If you're just starting, you might have to walk the mile or "jog-walk," and you might only be able to do a few repetitions of each of the three exercises. No problem. Do as few or as many of each as you can. But finish the circuit and you will have done a very effective mini-routine.

Now, want to ratch it up a notch or two?

Run the mile faster. See if you can do it in 10 minutes or under. Do a set of serious squats—20 reps, maybe with dumbbells or water bottles for added resistance. Don't rest. Go right to the push-ups. Try for 15. Go to the crunches. Twenty-five, in perfect form.

You can stop right there, or expand it even further by simply repeating the last three exercises: squats, push-ups, and crunches.

With a little imagination you can easily see how hard this workout can be (or how easy). More fit folk can run the mile faster, do more reps in each of the three exercises, and add another circuit of the last few. Heck, if you're truly a sucker for punishment, add another mile run when you're done with your last crunch.

It's simple, elegant, and very, very effective.

> Stress reduction is one of the best weight-loss strategies in the world. Stress can—and does—make you fat. Stress hormones cause cravings, overeating, and hormonal imbalances that lead to weight gain.

THE TO-DO LIST

THE TO-DO LIST

Keeping a to-do list is an important part of this program.

Each day you're going to make a list of actions or tasks that you've been putting off that would make a difference to you if you completed them. They can be small, easy actions, like returning a phone call or straightening up a closet. Or they can be significant, such as cleaning up a misunderstanding with a friend or parent that's been festering between the two of you for a long time. Don't get "stuck" on the meaning of the phrase "making a difference." To get a place on the list, an action doesn't have to be something gigantic like getting engaged or divorced or going back to school—but it *could* be. Sometimes just paying a phone bill or clearing out that old pile of Sunday newspapers near the bed creates a little whisper of mental fresh air that comes from finally doing something you've been putting off. There's no "right" way to make your list. Just do it. You're going to use this "master list" as one of your weekly assignments.

My To-Do List

Item	*Date Completed*
1. _____	_____
2. _____	_____
3. _____	_____
4. _____	_____
5. _____	_____
6. _____	_____
7. _____	_____
8. _____	_____
9. _____	_____
10. _____	_____
11. _____	_____

Item   **Date Completed**

12. _____   _____

13. _____   _____

14. _____   _____

15. _____   _____

16. _____   _____

17. _____   _____

18. _____   _____

19. _____   _____

20. _____   _____

21. _____   _____

22. _____   _____

23. _____   _____

24. _____   _____

25. _____   _____

26. _____   _____

27. _____   _____

28. _____   _____

29. _____   _____

30. _____   _____

31. _____   _____

32. _____   _____

33. _____   _____

34. _____   _____

35. _____   _____

36. _____   _____

37. _____   _____

38. _____   _____

39. _____   _____

40. _____   _____

41. _____   _____

42. _____   _____

Item	*Date Completed*
43. _____	_____
44. _____	_____
45. _____	_____
46. _____	_____
47. _____	_____
48. _____	_____
49. _____	_____
50. _____	_____
51. _____	_____
52. _____	_____
53. _____	_____
54. _____	_____
55. _____	_____
56. _____	_____
57. _____	_____
58. _____	_____
59. _____	_____
60. _____	_____

SELF-EVALUATION

SELF-EVALUATION

The Self-Evaluation Questions

One portion of each week's assignment is to write answers to a series of self-evaluation questions. Each week there are different questions. Answer them in the space provided. Don't think too much when you do this part—you might want to jot down the first thing that comes to mind. You can do this part of the week's assignment at any time during the week—you can work on it as the week goes on or you can even do it at the end of each week. If you haven't answered the questions for a given week when it's time to move to the next week, continue on to the next week anyway. You can always come back to the previous week's questions should you want to do so.

Why These Questions? Why These Exercises?

When people ask this question in seminars, I usually explain that these exercises are there partly to help you see that you are more than a number on the scale. When I say that, many people say, "But I *know* that already! I *know* who I am is not just my weight!" Some people even say, "I don't have to do all these airy-fairy exercises to prove that to myself. I just want some hard, cold techniques for losing weight!"

Fair enough. But it's rarely lack of technique and knowledge alone that keeps people from being all they want to be. No weight loss technique that is so narrowly focused as to include only things like portion size, percentage of calories from carbohydrates, and stuff like that is going to work unless you *also* deal with the things that come up in the exercises and questions. Believe me now, *those* are the things that sabotage you on your path. It's not for lack of understanding about the relationship of carbohydrates, insulin, and fat . . . I can explain that in a couple of chapters as I did in *Shape Up!*, and you'll know it, and that will be that. Lack of knowledge is not what's keeping you from being in shape. Sure, you need to have the knowledge, but that's the easy part—that's like having a map that tells you how to drive from California to New York. Lack of a map isn't what causes most people trouble on a journey—it's the unexpected things like bad weather, flat tires, engine trouble, distractions, money, running out of gas, hitting a tornado, getting discouraged and giving up . . . stuff like that. *That's* the stuff you need to be able to deal with to make your journey safely and successfully. Of course, the map is necessary—but it's the least significant part of what gets you where you want to go. Your skills for dealing with the *other* stuff are what make the most difference between winners and losers in this game (in fact, in most games in life, but that's a whole other discussion). Anyway, these exercises help you deal with the other stuff. These exercises help you learn about that car you're driving cross-country. In other words, you do these exercises to help you see who you really are and to examine who you are in a new way. When you have done that, you will be able to make the best use of the map that I've given you in *Shape Up!* and in this book.

In fact, you'll be able to draw your own map.

And that's really the point now, isn't it?

Optional

In the past decade, I've listened carefully to thousands of people I've been privileged to work with as well as hundreds of experts in fields ranging from weight loss to personal transformation that I've interviewed on my radio show, and if there's one single lesson I've taken away from all this listening, it's this: *Everything is related to everything.* The more you look into your life, the more you understand how everything fits together. The more you understand how everything fits together, the more power you have in the universe.

It's as simple as that.

With that simple truth in mind, I've put together some of the best "journaling" exercises I've found in the following section, "Exercises: Not the Physical Kind" (p.35). You don't have to do them, but you may find them fun, interesting, challenging, and enlightening.

Don't be surprised if connections begin to show up in areas of your life you didn't think had anything to do with your weight. Remember: It's *all* connected.

Enjoy the journey!

Exercises: Not the Physical Kind

Make a list of what you would like more of in your life.*

_____

_____

_____

_____

_____

_____

_____

_____

_____

_____

_____

Make a list of what you would like less of in your life.*

_____

_____

_____

_____

_____

_____

_____

_____

_____

_____

_____

(Hint: It might be interesting to visit this page from time to time during the eight-week program and see if you have any changes, additions, or subtractions to make)

*This exercise was donated by a good friend, the well-known personal coach and psychotherapist Roz Van Meter (wwwcoachroz.com). Used by permission.

Who are the most important people in your life?

_____

_____

_____

_____

_____

_____

_____

_____

Pick five of them and write down how you think they "see" you. Pick a few words that they might use to describe you or characterize their relationship to you.

1. *Person:* _____

   How he or she sees you: _____

   _____

   _____

   _____

   _____

   _____

2. *Person:* _____

   How he or she sees you: _____

   _____

   _____

   _____

   _____

   _____

3. *Person:* _____

   How he or she sees you: _____

   _____

   _____

_____
_____
_____

4. _Person:_ _____
   How he or she sees you: _____
   _____
   _____
   _____
   _____
   _____

5. _Person:_ _____
   How he or she sees you: _____
   _____
   _____
   _____
   _____
   _____

What would people most miss about you if you were gone?

_____
_____
_____
_____
_____
_____
_____
_____
_____
_____
_____
_____

The Anger Page

Who in your life are you angry at?

_____
_____
_____
_____
_____
_____

What would you like to say to that person that you have not been able to say?

_____
_____
_____
_____
_____
_____
_____
_____
_____
_____
_____
_____
_____
_____
_____
_____

Who could you not forgive?

_____
_____
_____
_____

What would it take for you to forgive that person?

_____

_____

_____

_____

_____

_____

_____

_____

_____

_____

What does it cost you to carry that anger around with you on a daily basis?

_____

_____

_____

_____

_____

_____

_____

_____

_____

_____

The Gratitude Page

List everything you have to be grateful for.

_____

_____

_____

_____

_____

_____

_____

_____

_____

_____

_____

_____

_____

_____

_____

_____

_____

_____

_____

_____

_____

_____

_____

_____

_____

_____

_____

_____

The following is a very difficult exercise and you may find it painful to do. It can be a very emotional experience. It's perfectly okay if you don't do it. However, many people have found that this exercise has opened the door to major breakthroughs in their lives.

If you do choose to do it, find a quiet place where you will be able to be alone and undisturbed. I recommend that you do this lying down, wearing comfortable clothes, with as few distractions as possible. You don't have to actually write down anything here unless you want to. I'd rather you simply lie down and think about these questions one by one. When you feel complete with the first question, move on to the second.

When you feel complete with the exercise on the first page, go on to the next page and spend some time thinking about the question you will see there.

The Second-Chance Exercise

Imagine that you have died. Actually visualize the scene of your own funeral. Who would be there? What would they be saying? What would they be doing? What would they be feeling? Spend a moment or two with each image, with each person. Stop right now and try to imagine this as vividly as possible. Do this before you go on to the next question. Then, consider each question carefully for as long as you need to before moving on to the next question.

What are the things you wish you had done that you never got to do?

What are the things that you wish you had said that you never got to say?

What are the things that now, on reflection, seem like they weren't so important?

What, if anything, do you wish you had done differently?

Is there anything now, on reflection, that you wished you had paid more attention to?

It's the end of your life. If you could go back in time and talk to *yourself* as you are right now, what would you tell yourself?

When you feel complete with this part of the exercise, go on to the next page.

What if you were given a second chance?

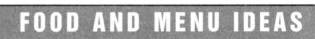

FOOD AND MENU IDEAS

FOOD AND MENU IDEAS

You'll have assignments each week to add and subtract foods using the following lists. You'll be adding foods to your diet from the "A" list, moderating or limiting foods from the "B" list, and watching the foods on the "C" list for individual reactions.

Food: Short Lists (for Quick Start)

"A" List

Vegetables: Spinach, alfalfa sprouts, okra, broccoli, collard greens, parsnips, cauliflower, cucumbers, kale, mushrooms, tomatoes, squash, snow peas, onions, peppers (all colors), brussel sprouts, cabbage, carrots, beets, celery, green beans, asparagus, turnips, fresh corn on the cob, eggplant, leeks, peas, chard, zucchini, artichokes, or any other vegetable—Also: Fresh vegetable juice!

Fish: All kinds

Eggs: Preferably organic, from free-range chickens

Meat: Preferably lean, antibiotic- and hormone-free, if available

Poultry: Chicken, turkey, preferably free-range

Protein powder: Whey is preferable, but soy is fine

Salads: All kinds; include some raw vegetables

Nuts: Almonds, pecans, walnuts, pistachio nuts, Brazil nuts, macadamias, raw cashews

Water: Purified or bottled

Fruit: Especially berries like blueberries, strawberries, raspberries, blackberries

Good fats: Extra-virgin olive oil, flaxseed oil, coconut, avocado, butter (small amounts)

Spices: Cinnamon, turmeric, ginger, rosemary, basil, mint, peppermint, spearmint, thyme, garlic, cayenne pepper, cloves, parsley, cumin seed

Tea: Green tea, black tea, herbal teas

"B List"

Commercial breads	Margarine
Bagels	Refined vegetable oils: Corn oil,
Pasta	sunflower oil, safflower oil, soy oil,
Cakes and pies	and other supermarket fare
Commercial dry cereals	Sugar
Packaged snack foods: Chips,	Sodas
candy bars, cupcakes,	Diet sodas
doughnuts, crackers, pretzels	Fruit juice

FOOD: Extended Lists

"A" List

Vegetables. Vegetables are the best things to add to your diet, and you can add them in unlimited amounts. Think in terms of color: Try to add every color to your shopping basket—red, orange, white, and especially green. Vegetables provide fiber, nutrients, antioxidants, phytochemicals, and enzymes in a low-calorie package, all of which helps you lose weight and gain health. Following is a partial list of vegetables to choose from. You can prepare them with olive oil or a little fresh creamy butter, and with as many seasonings as you like (see the list below for herbs and spices that are particularly recommended). Note: It's really important to include some raw foods on a daily basis for their enzyme content, so keep that in mind when adding vegetables to your diet.

> Rotate your food with the seasons. Foods in season are more in tune with the body's needs. For example, tropical fruits cool us in the summer; heavy soups sustain us in the winter.

Spinach	Alfalfa sprouts	Okra
Broccoli	Collard greens	Parsnips
Cauliflower	Cucumbers	Chard
Kale	Mushrooms	Zucchini
Snow Peas	Onions	Artichokes
Carrots	Peppers (all colors)	
Beets	Brussel sprouts	
Squash	Cabbage	
Green Beans	Celery	

Asparagus	Tomatoes
Turnips	Eggplant
Fresh corn on the cob	Leeks
Peas	

Water. Involved in every cellular process, water is the best weight-loss drink in the world. Forget the "eight glasses a day" recommendation and drink as much as you can, as often as you'd like. (Fruit juice and soda are not substitutes and coffee definitely doesn't count because, among other things, it's a diuretic.) You should make every effort to get pure, bottled, or filtered water.

Protein.

- Fish: In general, the more the better. If you can eat fish several times a week, that's great. One of the greatest health foods in the world is a can of sardines—and it's cheap, too! Following is a partial list of seafood from which to choose:

Tuna	Bluefish
Mackerel	Flounder
Whitefish	Yellowtail
Salmon	Mahi Mahi
Grouper	Scallops
Sardines	Shrimp

- Eggs: Eggs are one of nature's most perfect foods. They contain everything needed to support life. Eggs have been given a terrible rap in the popular press over the last decade, and as discussed at length in *Shape Up!* a very unfair one. Eat them and enjoy them, and this includes the yolks, which are a superb source of vitamin A and of phosphatidylcholine. Phosphatidylcholine is needed to form lecithin, which helps prevent cholesterol from being oxidized and is also a superb nutrient for liver health. Eggs also contain lutein and zeaxanthin, powerful carotenoids that are critical in protecting the eyes against macular degeneration. Dr. Fred Pescatore, author of *Feed Your Kids Right,* says, "If you buy one food that's organic, make it eggs." Organic eggs from free-range chickens are far more likely to contain a healthful amount of beneficial omega-3 fats, and some eggs now come with an "omega-3" guarantee on the box. Buy them!

- Whey Protein Powder: This is one of the most absorbable and bioavailable sources of protein on the planet, and it's inexpensive and versatile. Whey protein is also very immuno-protective, and causes the body to make more of one of its most critically important antioxidants, glutathione. It's great in shakes and can also be mixed with oatmeal. Shakes—especially made with whey protein—are a great way to get protein when you're crunched for time and can't sit down and eat.

- Meat: There is no inherent problem with eating meat, but the meat that is commonly available in supermarkets is unfortunately also a source of a lot of things we don't want, such as antibiotics, toxins, and hormones. To get all the benefits of meat and minimize the problems associated with it, you need to do some careful shopping. Veal and lamb are good choices, and so are the leanest cuts of Angus beef and any meat from animals that have been organically raised. The cuts from muscles that work hard are coarser in texture but have much less fat—examples are rump, eye of round, flank steak, and brisket. Whenever possible, try to get meat that is lean and antibiotic- and steroid-free. And don't rule out lean, trimmed, tender meats such as pork tenderloin and roast.

- Poultry: Free-range, antibiotic-free poultry is really worth the extra money if you can manage it.

Salads.   The addition of a salad a day, preferably before a meal, can do wonders for appetite management, not to mention the fiber, nutrients, phytochemicals, and antioxidants you'll be getting. Garnish with some nuts (see next item). By the way, this is also a great way to get some raw foods into your diet.

Nuts.   Nuts can be a great source of protein, essential fatty acids, and minerals. I'm not suggesting you sit and munch on handfuls of peanuts (which aren't a nut anyway, but a legume), but I *am* suggesting you include nuts in your diet on a regular basis. About a quarter cup is a good starting point for a portion. Pecans, almonds, walnuts, Brazil nuts, macadamia nuts, pistachios, and raw cashews are all fine. Try delicious nut butters (preferably organic) like almond, cashew, or even peanut, spread on a celery stick or half an apple.

With nuts, as with many foods, you have to be aware of your personal idiosyncratic reaction. Great as they may be, nuts are also subject to mold and rancidity, a definite problem for many people, especially people with candida. And some people are allergic to nuts. You can increase the odds of getting all the benefits by getting fresh, raw nuts and soaking them in water overnight, which makes them far more digestible. Sally Fallon, author of *Nourishing Traditions,* recommends draining them after an overnight soak and then toasting them in the oven on a baking sheet.

Fruit (Especially Berries).   Aim for up to two fruits a day, and choose from fruits lower in sugar like grapefruits, plums, apricots, apples, and pears and especially blueberries, raspberries, strawberries, and blackberries. They will give you healthful benefits without much problem from the standpoint of weight loss. This is not an "unlimited" item, though, because many fruits are high in sugar and eating too much fruit can create a scenario in your body that isn't conducive to weight loss. Ripe bananas, which are a staple of low-fat diet programs and that many people devour like candy, are a high-sugar item. Use with discretion!

Good Fats.   Olive oil: A couple of tablespoonfuls a day, preferably extra virgin and cold pressed, is a very good idea. It's even better if it's not heated (that is, use on salads or vegetables), but it is the preferred oil for cooking as well as eating.

Try to eat foods that are grown locally. Fruits and vegetables maintain their rich vitamin and phytonutrient content when they are eaten right after harvesting.

Other Good Fats: Most people who have been following the low-fat diet dogma are woefully underconsuming good fats. Paradoxically, some fats (like the omega-3 fats found in fish and flaxseed, and gamma-linolenic acid [GLA], a particular omega-6 fat found in evening primrose oil) can actually help you *lose* fat. These fatty acids kind of sit on the cell membrane and act as a cheerleader, encouraging other fats to get into the cell where they can be burned for fuel. Hopefully you learned in *Shape Up!* why the wholesale avoidance of fats was a very bad idea in the first place. The trick is to correct it by eating the *right* fats. Following is a partial list of fats—or foods that contain them—that you can begin to include in your diet:

- Flaxseed oil (but don't cook with it)
- Flaxseeds, ground (flaxseed meal)
- Avocados
- Nuts
- Nut butters
- Sesame Tahini
- Seeds
- Coconut
- Coconut oil
- Butter (in reasonable amounts)

And, of course, the fats found in cold-water fish such as salmon, tuna, mackeral, and sardines.

Spices and Herbs. Spices and herbs to use include cinnamon, turmeric, ginger, any leafy green herbs and plants in the mint family (for example, rosemary, basil, mint, peppermint, spearmint, thyme, and lemon balm), garlic (in all its forms), cayenne pepper, cloves, parsley, and cumin seed. Most of these herbs are loaded with antioxidants, and all of them have health-giving properties. Use herbs liberally and often.

Green Tea. Black tea has nearly as much antioxidant power as green tea, so you could use that as well.

Fresh Squeezed Vegetable Juice. Any kind, any combination.

"B" List

Commercial Breads. Most commercial breads have had all the good stuff processed out, even though many manufacturers attempt to make them "look" like warm and fuzzy health foods. Flour by definition is pulverized and defiberized grain and rarely has anything of benefit left in it. Most of the vitamins are lost in the processing. The manufacturer then throws a few paltry ones back in (hence the term "enriched"), which is rather like robbing the bank and leaving the bank tellers a few bucks for coffee. The only *possible* exception to the rule would be breads that are genuinely made with whole grains, but these are much harder to find than you would think, and definitely don't include most supermarket imposters. Get into the habit of reading the label for ingredients. Occasionally you will come across some breads that are actually made *without* flour—the ingredients will list, for example, "whole-grain rye, yeast, water, and salt," or seven different whole grains. (One of the best, though it's an acquired taste, is Eziekel bread.) In addition, most breads are highly glycemic, and can provoke a high insulin response—not a good thing. For that reason, I think it's a good idea to really limit bread, at least for a while, and see how you feel. Breads are also very easy to overeat.

Be aware that many people have food sensitivities to gliadin, a fraction of gluten that is found mainly in wheat but also in many other grains. This sensitivity may not be a full-blown allergy, but it can show up as symptoms ranging from water retention and bloating to headaches, weight gain, and "brain fog." More people than you might imagine have this sensitivity, and if you are one of them, any grain that contains gluten, and definitely any wheat product, is going to be a problem for you. This includes couscous (which is just tiny pasta) and tabouli (which is just cracked wheat). Many people are amazed at how good they feel when they remove wheat from their diet. You may not be one of them, but it's definitely worth finding out if you are. If you're not ready to go all the way and eliminate wheat for a period of time, you might want to experiment by seriously reducing your consumption or by trying gluten-free grains. Some "halfway house" alternatives that are a big improvement over commercial wheat products include polenta or cornbread, provided you make it with a whole-grain cornmeal (like Arrowhead Mills™). Remember, though, that these are still high-carbohydrate, high-calorie items that should come with a "handle with care" label.

Bagels.   Contrary to popular belief, bagels are anything but a health food. They contain the worst of everything that's wrong with bread, plus, caloriewise, they cost a pretty penny. If you must indulge, scoop out the doughy, yeasty middle part and eat the crust, preferably with some nut butter, turkey, or salmon.

Commercial Pasta.   Virtually everything true of breads (above) is also true of pasta. In addition, the portions we commonly consume of this food are simply outrageous.

If you're not ready to give it up completely, that's fine—but use it as a small side dish. Load it up with vegetables and add some protein and a little olive oil. Don't make it a main dish, and don't consume it often.

Cakes and Pies. This category also includes desserts, doughnuts, and any other packaged little cakes or cupcakes.

Commercial Cereals. Sadly, this includes virtually everything on the supermarket shelf that comes in a box with a cute little picture on it. The good news is that it doesn't include oatmeal, buckwheat groats (kasha), and whole-grain grits. These are "good" starches. The same caveats about breads apply here, though—don't over-consume.

Packaged Snack Foods. Chips, candy bars, cupcakes, doughnuts, crackers, and yes, pretzels too.

Refined Vegetable Oils. This is one of the worst items on the list. Don't eat them or cook with them. I'm talking about virtually every common supermarket oil *including* canola, which has been falsely marketed as healthy because it contains some omega-3 fats—(however, that very fact makes it a bad choice for cooking). If you can find cold-pressed, organic canola oil, that would be okay, but even then I wouldn't heat it to high temperatures. Avoid refined corn oil, sunflower oil, safflower oil, soy oil, and other supermarket fare like the plague. If you really need these oils, it is truly worth making the trip to the health food store and spending the extra money for cold-pressed, unrefined oils that have not been damaged by processing with high heat and chemicals. Remember, even the "best" vegetable oils are still mostly omega-6's and heavy reliance on them exacerbates the imbalance between the omega-6's that we overconsume and the omega-3's that we underconsume. Experiment with alternative sources like flax, sesame, pistachio, walnut, hazelnut, and grapeseed. Get the best quality you can find and mix and match your fats. Use extra-virgin (cold-pressed) olive oil whenever possible. Reasonable amounts of fresh butter are fine, and for cooking, use peanut or coconut oil.

Margarine.   Margarine is one of the stupidest mistakes ever made by the food industry, a virtual orgy of trans-fatty acid orgy. It's a disgrace that some of the establishment groups actually endorsed this stuff as "heart healthy." Go back to butter.

Sugar.   Sugar may be the hardest food to give up (you may have to do it gradually), but to the extent that you can do it, you will experience profound and dramatic results both in weight loss and general health. Remember, table sugar is only the most obvious form; there are about nineteen other disguises in which it sneaks into our food. The more sugar-sensitive you are, the more on guard you need to be.

Sodas.   A neat little package of sugar, calories, chemicals, and caffeine, and a calcium robber if ever there was one. Not one good thing about it, unless you're comparing it with heroin.

Diet Sodas.   The evidence is overwhelming that they don't help you lose weight at all, and the evidence is compelling that they do you more harm than good.

Fruit Juice.   This is a pure sugar hit, and definitely not a health food. It has little of the good stuff in the fruit, and no fiber to slow the effect on blood sugar and insulin levels. If you make your own with a blender like Vita-Mix™ or even a juicer, it's better than the commercial kind, but even then, I still recommend that you do home-made mixes that favor vegetables and use a smaller amount of fruit. The only exception to the store-bought fruit juice rule would be unsweetened cranberry juice, which is hard to find, very tart, and rather expensive. However, it provides a lot of digestive enzymes and when diluted with water makes a nice morning drink.

"C" List

There are a number of foods that are just very problematic for some people, whereas others seem to be able to do fine with them. I've put these foods on a third short list, the "C" list. My suggestion is to monitor your reaction to them very carefully and decide whether they fit into your strategy at all, and if so, to what extent.

Wheat.   Wheat is a source of food reactions and sensitivities that go undetected for many people. Until they try taking it out of their diet for a while, many people don't realize how much wheat affects them. Wheat is also in virtually every processed food on the market, so if you remove it from your diet you're also getting rid of a lot of junk. It's definitely an ingredient worth monitoring—you might not be one of the many people in the world who actually do better on a wheat-free diet, but if you are in doubt, taking wheat out of your diet for a week or two might be a revelation.

Starches.   In general, it is easy to overeat starches—keep an eye on quantities. If fat loss is a goal, you will probably have to choose them very carefully and limit the portion sizes. However, that said, there *is* a short list of starches that are great health foods. My favorites are sweet potatoes (or yams), oatmeal (not the instant kind, but the steel-cut, slow-cooking type), lentils, chickpeas, and most beans. Whole-grain grits and buckwheat groats (kasha) are acceptable as well. Rice has a low allergen potential (unlike many other grains) but is a food high in starch that can easily sabotage weight loss. Try brown rice or basmati for variety. Many people find that one to two starches a day is a good place to begin while you figure out your best strategy.

Milk.   I do not believe supermarket milk is a good food for adults or children. Homogenization changes the nature of the fat, pasteurization destroys the enzymes, the protein in milk (casein) is a major allergen, most of the world is lactose intolerant, and dairy foods are extremely mucous forming for a large segment of the population. The wholesale use of bovine growth hormone to increase milk production troubles me greatly. I have no objection to raw, certified milk (if you can find it) or organic milk from a small family farm, but in my opinion modern processing has taken what once might have been a very healthy food (for some, anyway) and turned it into something that it is very difficult to recommend for anyone. In fairness, some people seem to do fine with milk, but enough people have told me that their lives have changed (and their weight-loss plateaus ended) when they eliminated dairy products (and/or wheat) for me to recommend that you at least consider removing it for a while to see if it makes a difference.

Other Dairy Foods.   Dairy food is not for all people, but there are some people who tolerate it better than others. For those people, cottage cheese and other soft cheeses like feta and farmer's can be treated as "A" list foods. Goat cheese is superb. Even hard cheeses for those who tolerate them are fine on occasion, particularly Swiss, a great source of calcium. If you're buying hard cheeses, look for those made from raw milk. If you even suspect a yeast problem, avoid the fermented kind like bleu cheese and roquefort. Yogurt is fine as long as it's *not* the no-fat kind, which is loaded with sugar, and as long as it has real live cultures. If you can find them, sheep milk and goat milk varieties of yogurt taste great and are extremely nutritious. So are naturally fermented dairy products like kefir.

Coffee. Coffee is an adrenal stimulant and as such releases sugar into the bloodstream. It also triggers stress hormones, which can ultimately cause weight gain and adrenal burnout. If you can live without coffee, great. If you can't, you can definitely do "damage control" on this one and continue to enjoy it from time to time by reducing the amount you consume, switching to organic, grinding your own beans, and using unbleached filters and filtered water.

Alcohol. To drink or not to drink is a personal decision, but alcohol has sabotaged more weight-loss plans than you can shake a diet book at. Alcohol not only relaxes social inhibitions but eating inhibitions too. Moderate is the operative word here. For some people "moderation" is a perfectly acceptable strategy. For others, "moderation" might as well be a word in a foreign language that your brain simply doesn't recognize. Only *you* can know which category you belong in.

A Word About Soy. Anybody who claims to have the final answer on soy at this point in time is standing on quicksand.

There are many good things in real soy products, but some very smart people in the field of nutrition have raised some doubts about the wholesale marketing of soy as the answer to all our nutritional prayers. With the current state of the debate, I think the most prudent position for now is the one taken by the journal *Alternative Medicine:*

- try to get your soy products from non–genetically modified sources;
- whenever possible eat naturally fermented products like miso and tempeh or real beans in the edame form;

- don't rely on soy as your sole source of protein unless you are a strict vegan;
- don't take concentrated supplements of soy isoflavones.

The Shape Up plan was never designed to dictate meal plans to you—in fact, that's completely counter to the spirit of the program, which is one of the things that sets it apart from so many other diets. But in recognition of the fact that many people find themselves out of whack when it comes to food, confused about nutritional do's and don'ts, fatigued, running on empty, relying on artificial stimulants like caffeine and sugar to get through the day, and frustrated with their inability to "get motivated and get started," I've put together a kind of "training wheels" program to get you going. Understand that this is a guide. You can mix and match and customize to your heart's content. All I ask is that you do so consciously. Pay attention to the effect that changes in your food—and its timing—has, not just on your weight but on your overall sense of well-being.

Remember: on the Shape Up program, you're only "cheating" when you're not paying attention. Food is information—learn from your eating and you'll be well on your way to success.

Shopping List

Blueberries and/or raspberries (frozen if you can't get fresh)
Dried cranberries
Whey protein powder (or soy protein powder) or preferably both
Pineapple juice (optional)
Grapefruit
Apples
Nut butter: almond (best), peanut (perfectly okay); organic is preferable
Dates or raisins
Oatmeal (not the instant kind)
Almonds, walnuts, or pecans
Coconut for sprinkling
Whole-grain or gluten-free bread (for those who aren't ready to try bread-free)
Free-range eggs, omega-3 rich if you can find them

Meat, fish, or poultry (for dinners, lunches)

Vegetables: peppers, mushrooms, onions, tomatoes, and so on, the more the better, every possible color and every possible variety (see suggestions under "Dinner," below)

Starchy vegetables: sweet potatoes, basmati rice, corn on the cob, and so forth (see suggestions under "Dinner")

Shape-Up Friendly?

All of these meals are extremely Shape-Up friendly. Notice that some of them do contain dairy products, and some contain bread. Why? Because the whole premise of Shape Up, which can't be repeated often enough, is that *everybody's different.* There is no doubt left in my mind after doing this for ten years that there are an untold number of people on the planet who feel indescribably better when they eliminate dairy, wheat, or both from their diet, but there is also no doubt in my mind that this doesn't apply to everyone. The whole Shape-Up program is respectful not only of these individual dietary and metabolic differences, but of the fact that different people need to approach dietary changes at different rates of speed. Shape Up is about you finding your own road in your own time frame. If you're currently eating a standard bacon and eggs and toast and juice and sausage breakfast, a switch to Dr. Baker's Special Shake might be a bit much, but a switch to vegetable omelette or eggs any style with gluten-free toast might be just the ticket. If you can't even think about giving up bread or cereal, why not just improve the quality of these foods and the effect they have on your blood sugar and insulin levels with a gentle, not-too-radical move to half a grapefruit with gluten-free toast, almond butter, and yogurt or with cereal, milk, and an egg?

The goals:

- Eat low glycemic carbohydrates that don't raise blood sugar quickly (the ones listed all qualify).
- Concentrate on protein and good fats during the day and save most of your carbohydrates (especially starchy carbs) for late afternoon/evening.
- Eat breakfast like a king, lunch like a prince, and dinner like a pauper.
- When in doubt, go for real foods and pure water.

The body's biochemcial rhythms require protein during the day and carbohydrates at night. This seems to go against "conventional wisdom"—that is, the idea that you need high carbohydrates during the day for "energy"—but the fact is that *protein should be emphasized during the day and that you should consume most of your carbohydrates in the evening.* That's not a license to down huge amounts of pasta and bread at dinner and late-night popcorn and pretzels—to lose weight and feel great you still need to stick with the "good" carbs and consume them moderately (personally, I believe that only in rare cases should carbohydrates constitute more than 40 percent of your diet). What I'm saying shouldn't be taken to mean you eat *nothing* but protein during the day and *nothing* but carbs at night—we're talking *emphasis* here. Again, your individual circumstances will dictate to what degree you can make the switch. All of the suggested breakfasts contain good proteins.

Breakfast

1. Dr. Sid Baker's Special Shake: 3 ounces of milk, 3 ounces of yogurt, 1 scoop of soy or whey protein, 1 tablespoon (or more) ground flaxseeds (flax meal), ¼ cup blueberries (or raspberries or blackberries), and ice

2. Special Shake/variation: substitute 6 ounces of rice milk for the 3 ounces of milk and 3 ounces of yogurt in the above recipe

3. Jonny's Favorite: 1 scoop of soy or whey protein, 6–8 ounces of water, 2 tablespoons of oatmeal, 1 tablespoon of almond (or peanut) butter, flax meal, and ice

4. Jonny's Favorite (variation): 1 scoop of soy or whey protein, 3–4 ounces of pineapple juice, 3–4 ounces of water, and flax meal

5. Homemade Wrap: Quick-stir-fry chicken, tomatoes, and peppers and wrap in a large lettuce leaf. Sprinkle with extra-virgin olive oil after cooking, or with blended oil

6. Vegetable Omelette: Make an omelette using 2–3 eggs with mushrooms, peppers, tomatoes, and onions (a small amount of cheese is optional) (optional: half a grapefruit is perfectly fine)

7. Eggs: 2–3 eggs any style and one slice of gluten-free toast

8. Eggs: 2–3 eggs any style and oatmeal with 1 pat butter or 2 tablespoons of half-and-half or cream (or mix ½ pat butter with 1 tablespoon half-and-half or cream)

9. Vegetable Omelette: Eggs with mushrooms, onions, peppers, and tomatoes (optional: one slice of gluten-free toast)

On the Go

1. Half a grapefruit, one slice of gluten-free toast,* 1 tablespoon of almond butter, and 3 ounces of yogurt

2. Half a grapefruit, a small bowl of whole-grain, high-fiber cereal (at least 5 grams of fiber per serving), a sprinkle of coconut, soy or regular milk, and 1 hard- or soft-boiled egg

3. Homemade Muesli: Presoak 2–3 ounces of slow-cooking oats plus 1 ounce of raisins or dates, 1 ounce of almonds, and a sprinkle of coconut with 3 ounces or so of soy milk till soft; 1 hard- or soft-boiled egg (Packs up nicely in a plastic container.)

4. Travel Special: Yogurt (not the no-fat kind), 1 ounce of almonds, and 2 ounces of farmer's cheese or other cheese. Optional: a hard-boiled egg. (This breakfast is a cinch to pack up "to go.") Optional: Take along some berries or a small apple.

For those who are interested, the calorie content of all of these meals is in the 300–400 range (some a drop less, some a drop more). Overall, the exact calorie count is *far less* important than the quality of the food and the fact that these meals will not put you into blood sugar hell and insulin overdrive. They will sustain your energy throughout the morning (if you need a snack, see below) and once you find the ones that work best for you, you will find that you feel better than you have in a long time.

Remember also that although you can follow these recipes and meal plans to the letter, it is also perfectly okay to use them as templates, and to mix and match. For example, if the taste of plain protein powder with water and ice doesn't bother you,

you can use it as a substitute for the hard- or soft-boiled egg in the cereal-based breakfasts (half a grapefruit, whole-grain, high-fiber cereal, milk, and a hard- or soft-boiled egg or Homemade Muesli).

A note on time saving: Most of these breakfasts can be prepared a lot quicker than you might think. If you are *absolutely positive* that these are too time-consuming and you are *sure* they wouldn't fit into your lifestyle (kids, school, and so on), consider the following radical proposition (bear with me now): How about changing your lifestyle slightly? Sitting down to breakfast, having it with family, structuring the morning so that the kids actually have to eat before leaving for school, spending just a little time lovingly preparing fresh food together (or even for yourself)—all can have amazing benefits in everyone's overall health, well-being, stress reduction, and sense of relatedness and community. I know it sounds radical, but consider it for a moment. When we talk about "lifestyle" changes as opposed to just "diet," this is what we mean!

> When it comes to food, think proactively. If you know you're going to be stuck in a situation where you're going to be hungry and there's only going to be junk food available, plan ahead: bring along some nuts and dried fruit.

Lunch

1. Chicken breast without skin and a green salad
2. Tuna with mixed vegetables
3. Lean beef with mixed vegetables
4. Steamed chicken and broccoli
5. Sardines and a green salad
6. Turkey and peppers
7. Chili and vegetables

(Fresh vegetable soup can be added to any of the above.)

Select Recipes

Breakfast

Paleo-Shake

1 scoop PaleoMeal Powder*
1 tablespoon organic almond butter
1 cup blueberries (fresh or frozen)
4 ice cubes
6–8 oz pure filtered water

*I recommend Paleomeal whey protein powder by Designs for Health because it not only tastes good and is very high quality, but it also has additional omega-3 fats, lecithin, and other important nutrients. You can order it at 1–800-847-8302 or on my website at www.jonnybowden.com. . . If you prefer you can substitute any good quality whey protein powder, or, if you like, you can use soy protein.

Homemade Museli and One Hard-Boiled Egg

The Museli

___ cup raw, uncooked oats (not the instant kind), add 8–9 almonds, a dozen raisins. Cover with enough goats milk (or soy milk) to moisten well. Season with cinnamon, sweeten with blackstrap molasses to taste (or use raw unfiltered honey). Eat when soft enough to be chewy but not soggy

Bodybuilders Special: Easy Oatmeal and Eggs

Cover ___ cup of raw, uncooked oats with ___ oz pure filtered water. In a separate bowl, scramble one egg, add the egg to oatmeal, add a little pure filtered water to make oatmeal/egg mixture moist. Sprinkle with sliced almonds, microwave the mix for four minutes. After cooking, moisten further with goats or soy milk and mix to desired consistency (stiff or creamy). Top with a $\frac{1}{2}$ pat of butter (or a little flax oil), season with cinnamon. Sprinkle with some flax seeds, sweeten if necessary with blackstrap molasses or pure unfiltered honey.

Shape-Up Pancake

1 egg (preferably organic, free range)

$\frac{1}{4}$ cup ground almonds (or $\frac{1}{8}$ cup ground almonds and $\frac{1}{8}$ cup ground cashews)

$\frac{1}{4}$ cup goats milk (or soy milk)

cinnamon to taste

Mix ingredients together, cook as regular pancake on a preheated griddle or fry pan well moistened with olive oil or butter.

Traditional Toast Made Better

1 tablespoon organic (raw or toasted) almond butter

1 slice toasted sprouted whole grain bread

3 oz whole yogurt (goats milk is a great variety)

3 oz goats or soy milk (organic cows milk OK for those who tolerate it)

Top the toast with the almond butter; you can spread the yogurt on top, or eat separately.

The Ultimate Vegetable Omlette

$\frac{1}{2}$ red or yellow bell pepper (diced or sliced)

$\frac{1}{2}$ green pepper (diced or sliced)

$\frac{1}{2}$ cup mushrooms (diced or sliced)

$\frac{1}{2}$ medium red onion (sliced)

1 cup tomato (sliced)

4 eggs (organic, free range)

Scramble eggs, set aside. Heat skillet with butter; sautee the onions till transparent, add peppers, mushrooms, tomato. Add the scrambled eggs, sprinkle with cheddar cheese while cooking (optional). Scramble to desired consistency, season with salt and pepper and serve.

Lunch

Cassandra and Jonny's Blueberry Salad

$^{1}/_{2}$ – $^{3}/_{4}$ cup of blueberries

6–8 small, bite-sized squares of swiss cheese OR

crumble or shred 2 oz of goat cheese

2 cups of spinach leaves (or arugula or mescalin mix)

$^{1}/_{4}$ cup tamari almonds

1 cup cherry tomatoes

$^{1}/_{4}$ small-medium avocado, sliced or diced

Toss salad together with *unrefined* toasted sesame oil (Spectrum Oils) or extra-virgin olive oil (approx. 2 tablespoons). Sprinkle with flax seeds.

Easy High-Protein Lunch

1 can sardines (in olive oil, water, or tomato sauce)

1 large tomato, sliced

2 or 3 thin slices of mozarella cheese (or equivalent feta amount feta)

1 medium-sized red (or green) bell pepper, sliced

Arrange the slices of tomato, pepper, and cheese, alternating (with the cheese in the middle for color). Use 1 tablespoon of olive oil, squeezed lemon, and salt and pepper to season. Eat with sardines.

Fast-Food Lunch Made Better

2 cups mescalin mix (or arugula)

$^{1}/_{4}$ cup anchoives (or anchoive paste to taste)

3 ounces chicken diced (about $^{1}/_{2}$ cup)

cherry tomatoes, sliced bell pepper

Toss salad and top with extra-virgin olive oil, salt and pepper, and seasoning.

or:

Order chicken caesar salad from food court. Take out croutons; add cherry tomatoes if available, use olive oil dressing.

Cassandra's Special Tuna

1 6 oz can of tuna in water (Starkist™ or equivalent)
2 tablespoons of honey mustard
$\frac{1}{2}$ cup cherry tomatoes
$\frac{1}{3}$ cup almond slivers
$\frac{1}{4}$ cup diced onion (red or white) (optional)
$\frac{1}{3}$ cup diced celery (optional)
Serve on a bed of lettuce, or wrap in a lettuce leaf.

Fast and Delicious Homemade Melt

4 oz sliced turkey from the deli (fresh turkey is always better if you can
    get it)
2 slices swiss cheese
2 cups baby spinach leaves or mixed arugula greens
1 dozen raisins
Arrange the turkey on a plate, cover with the swiss cheese, sprinkle on
the raisins and put in microwave until swiss cheese melts (different on
different microwaves—about a minute). Put the spinach leaves or mixed
greens on a plate, and arrange the turkey/cheese on top.

Dinner

Shape-Up Baked Vegetable Chicken

boneless, skinless chicken (1 piece for each person) (you can cook with
    skin and discard skin after cooking)
mixed vegetables of any kind: broccoli, cauliflower, spinach, kale, carrots
are all good (allow about 2 cups of mixture per person)
1 chopped onion
1 large sliced tomato (or equivalent in cherry tomatos)
$\frac{1}{4}$ cup sliced almonds
parsley to taste

oregano to taste

pepper to taste

Put a large piece of foil on a large cookie sheet. Place chicken in middle and top with vegetables, olive oil, and seasonings. Seal the foil tight leaving a little space inside for steaming. Bake for 30 minutes @ 400 degrees. Take out of oven and add the tomatoes, onions, and almonds. Seal again and finish baking for about 10 minutes. Open the top of the foil for another 5–10 minutes if the chicken was frozen to begin with.

Jonny's Steamed Vegetables and Sweet Potato

Steamed Vegetables

1 onion, sliced

2 cups broccoli florets (you can substitute stringbeans)

1 cup carrots, cut into 1–2 inch pieces

1 red, orange, or yellow bell pepper, sliced

Mix vegetables and steam in a wooden steamer. When still brightly colored but slightly softened, arrange on plate. Top with 1 pat of butter per person; salt, pepper, lemon, and spices to taste. Serve with $1/2$ medium or 1 small baked sweet potato, topped with $1/2$ pat butter and 1 tablespoon flax oil. Season potato with cinnamon

Note: this is a vegetarian meal, suitable for dinner. If you want protein with it, simply add a cup of diced tofu to the vegetable mixture while steaming.)

Baked Salmon Fillet

Salmon fillet or steak (approx 4. ounces per person)

Juice of 1 orange

3 teaspoons extra-virgin olive oil

lemon-pepper spice (or fish seasoning spice)

1 or 2 small lemons

Arrange the salmon in a baking pan that has a lid. Mix olive oil and orange juice together and brush over the salmon. Sprinkle with the spice (lemon-pepper, or fish seasoning). Cut up the lemon into slices and arrange over the fish as garnish. Bake at 350 for 15–25 minutes until done.

(Can be served with any vegetable dish, salad, basmati rice, or combination.)

Shape-Up Almond Butter Chicken

4 large boneless, skinless chicken breasts

1 medium size onion

$1/3$ cup almond butter

3 tablespoon olive oil, divided

3 tablespoon lemon juice, divided

$1/2$ teaspoon ground cumin

$1/4$ teaspoon salt

$1/4$ teaspoon garlic powder

$1/2$ cup pure filtered water

Make a marinade by combining 2 tbs oil, 2 tablespoons lemon juice, salt and cumin. Add chicken and marinate 10 minutes. Broil chicken until tender. Turn as needed. Meanwhile: heat 1 tablespoon olive oil over medium heat. Saute the onion in the olive oil till golden or transparent; add in the water, the garlic powder, and 1 tablespoon of the lemon juice. Bring the mixture to a boil and remove from heat. Beat in the almond butter until melted. Pour over the chicken and serve warm.

Goes great with any salad (including beet and orange salad below) or steamed vegetables.

Shape-Up Beet and Orange Salad with Chicken Breast

Beet and Orange Salad

2 cups sliced beets, cooked and drained

3 tablespoons cider vinegar (apple cider vinegar is also fine)

$1/4$ cup chopped red onion

$^1/_4$ teaspoon ground cumin

green leaf lettuce

1 teaspoon raw unfiltered honey (optional)

2 large oranges, peeled, sectioned

Make marinade by putting vinegar, cumin, and honey (optional) in a non-staining bowl and stiring till well-mixed. Add beets and onion and stir gently till they're well coated with the marinade. Refrigerate for at least an hour. Line a plate with lettuce leaves. Remove the beets and onions from the marindade with a slotted spoon and place in the middle of the plate. Encircle them with the orange wedges.

Serve with 1 baked chicken breast (cold or hot) or with Almond Butter Chicken (above).

Snacks

1. Jonny's Favorite: Blueberries, cherry tomatoes, 2 ounces of Swiss cheese cubed, and half a dozen almonds (optional: sprinkle with oil*)

2. Cassandra's Favorite: A handful of dried cranberries, a handful of tamari almonds, a handful of cubed farmer's cheese (or other hard cheese made from raw milk), and a handful of cherry tomatoes

3. Raw sliced peppers and tomatoes (optional but recommended: drizzle with oil*)

4. Blueberries, cherry tomatoes, and 1 ounce of almonds (optional: sprinkle with oil)*

5. Half a sweet potato (prebaked) (yes, they're delicious cold) with turkey slices (recommended for later in the day)

6. One can of sardines and cherry tomatoes on red leaf lettuce

7. Apple slices spread with almond or peanut butter

8. One or 2 ounces of almonds, pistachio nuts, Brazil nuts, macadamia nuts, pecans, or walnuts

9. Celery sticks spread with almond or peanut butter

10. A can of tuna packed in water with celery and onion (optional: 1 table-spoon of homemade mayo, but make it with organic eggs and extra-virgin olive oil, *or* sprinkle with oil)*

11. Sliced tomatoes and 2 ounces of farmer's cheese or other cheese; sprinkle with oil*

12. Four turkey slices with sliced tomatoes (optional: sprinkle tomatoes with oil*)

13. Leftover beef slices with sliced tomatoes (optional: sprinkle tomatoes with oil*)

14. Real yogurt (not the no-fat kind) with 1 ounce of almonds

*Extra-virgin olive oil, flaxseed oil, Essential Woman™, Omega Balance™, or Udo's Choice™

Dinner

Choose one food from column A, one from column B, and one from column C

A (3–4 oz portion)	**B** (generous helping)	**C** (starchy carbs)
Salmon	Spinach	Sweet potato
Tuna	Kale	Corn on the cob
Grouper	Asparagus	Lentils
Mackerel	Artichokes	Beans
Sardines	Bok choy	Basmati rice
Any other fish on	Broccoli	Chickpeas
the fish list (p. 47)	Collards	Peas
Beef	Cauliflower	Whole-grain bread (1 slice)
Lamb	Brussel sprouts	Barley
Chicken	Carrots	
Turkey		
Cabbage		
Pumpkin		
Squash		
Tomatoes		
Peppers		
Eggplants		
Onions		
Leeks		
Beets		
Cucumbers		
Any other vegetable on		
the vegetable list (page 46)		

The following is a chart of the glycemic index of some representative foods. The glycemic index is a relative measure of how quickly a food, eaten by itself, will raise your blood sugar. This version of the index uses white bread, which is rated at 100, as the measuring standard.

Cherries	32	Pastry	84
Lentils	36	Cheese pizza	86
Grapefruit	36	Ice cream	87
Pearled barley	36	Hamburger bun	87
Kidney beans	42	High-fructose corn syrup	89
Butter beans	44	Beets	91
Dried apricots	44	Macaroni and cheese	92
Chocolate milk	49	Wheat bread	97
Pears	53	Stonewheat Thins	96
Apples	54	Cream of Wheat	100
Plums	55	Potato boiled/mashed	104
Grapes	66	Whole-wheat snack bread	105
Green peas	68	Doughnut	108
Mixed-grain bread	69	Waffles	109
Carrots	70	Instant potatoes	118
Oatmeal	70	Cornflakes	119
Yams	73	Instant rice	128
Sweet corn	78	Malodextrin	150
Brown rice	79	Tofu nondairy frozen dessert	164
White rice	83		

Remember: Not all high-glycemic foods are "bad" and not all low-glycemic foods are "good." However, keeping the glycemic index in mind can help you to create meals that are not heavily weighted toward the high end of the scale. That will go a long way toward keeping you off the blood-sugar roller coaster and keeping energy levels even and cravings at bay.

Top Ten Things to Think About When Shopping in Supermarkets

1. *Shop the outer edges of the market.* The periphery is where the good stuff is concentrated; everything comes in packages in the middle aisles.

2. *If you can't pronounce the ingredients, be suspicious.* The more ingredients something contains, the more it is a "food product" and the less it is a food. Only real food belongs in your shopping cart.

3. *Shop for color.* It can take years of study to memorize all the carotenoids, flavonoids, antioxidants, phytochemicals, and other wonderful stuff found in fruits and vegetables but it's relatively simple to put together a food basket that looks like an art project. Get as many colors in there as possible—red, yellow, orange, and especially green—and you'll cover all the bases.

4. *Don't fear meat.* But look for lean cuts, and start demanding antiobiotic- and hormone-free or free-range meat. Meat and eggs are only as good as the lives of the animals that gave them to us. If an animal lived in a box where it couldn't move for most of its life and was force-fed grains and fattened with hormones and steroids, how good do you think it's going to be for the person who eats it? How nice it would be if we could go back to thinking like the American Indians and respecting and honoring the animals we eat for food, and how much healthier it would be for us as well. Something to think about.

5. *Read labels.* Don't buy something unless you know what's in it, and this means looking at a lot more than how many grams of fat it has.

6. *Look for the sugar content.* It's listed under "total carbohydrates" on every label. Four grams of sugar equals one teaspoon of sugar. Think about that the next time you pick up a box of cereal.

7. *Look for the fiber content.* The more the better. If you're buying cereal, try for five grams or more.

8. *Look for the term "hydrogenated" or "partially hydrogenated" oil.* If you see it, run the other way. This won't be easy, because the food industry fills most packaged goods—cakes, pastries, crackers, cookies, and cereals—with the stuff, but start being aware of it and avoid it as much as possible. "Partially hydrogenated" means it's loaded with possibly the most damaging class of fat, "trans-fatty acids."

9. *Don't buy refined oils.* Another difficult one, I know, especially with all the healthy sounding labels that proclaim "no cholesterol" or "all-vegetable." Don't be fooled. Refined "cooking" oils have all the good stuff removed from them, like the natural antioxidant vitamin E, and contain virtually no omega-3 fats. The food industry loves this stuff because it can sit on the shelf forever without spoiling, but just for your information, rats won't even go near it. That should tell you something!

10. *Think "Caveman."* I know it's hard in today's modern world, but make a game of it. Pretend you were just transported into the future (today) from an earlier time when you were a hunter-gatherer and lived on and by the land. See what foods in your supermarket might look familiar to your hunter-gatherer psyche. Buy those.

> Fat-free is neither healthy nor wise. Fats are essential to human health. They are the raw materials from which important substances in the body are made, and some of them can actually *help* you lose body fat.

WEEK ONE

WEEK ONE

Optimists are right. So are pessimists.
It's up to you to choose which you will be.

—HARVEY MACKAY

Food Goals

- Three meals per day with beginnings and endings.
- No standing in front of the fridge, no mindless eating, no "sampling" of whatever is there. Mindfulness is the key word.
- Keep a thorough record of everything you eat. Notice any connections to mood and energy. This week the main element you are adding is *consciousness*.
- Eat at least *one food* from the "A" list on a daily basis.

Exercise Goals

- Beginners: Walking for ten minutes a day, three times this week
- Intermediates: Cardio four times a week for twenty to thirty minutes
- Advanced: Cardio five times a week for thirty to forty-five minutes (group fitness classes can be substituted for cardio workout, and so can a fitness video)

Most overeating is unconscious. Use this workbook as a tool to pay attention to what you're eating and to discover the relationship between what you eat and what you feel.

To-Do List Goals

- Expand the list and add any new items you think of that feel like they belong on the list.
- Do at least two tasks from the master to-do list. Any two. Check them off when you complete them, and enter them in the Week One Round-Up. (Hint: no item is too insignificant. It all counts.)

Day One: _____

(fill in your personal start date, for example Monday, January 1)

Goals for Today

_____

_____

_____

Food Record

_____

_____

_____

_____

_____

_____

_____

_____

_____

Exercise Today

_____

_____

_____

_____

_____

_____

_____

_____

Which "A" list food was added to today's menu?

_____

End-of-the-Day Questions

1. What kind of day did you have? _____
2. What was your energy like? _____
3. Notice any connections between food and mood? Between food and energy? Between food and feelings? _____
4. Any comments about what you liked or didn't like about your day? Did you come up against any obstacles today? What were they? *Who* were they? _____
   _____
5. Any final thoughts or feelings or things you need to say to complete the day for yourself?
   _____
   _____
   _____
6. Can you let what happened today be the way it was and be the way it was not? (Either a simple "yes" or "no" is okay.) _____

Day Two: _____

Goals for Today

_____

_____

_____

Food Record

_____

_____

_____

_____

_____

_____

_____

_____

Exercise Today

_____

_____

_____

_____

_____

_____

_____

_____

_____

Which "A" list food was added to today's menu?

_____

End-of-the-Day Questions

1. What kind of day did you have? _____

2. What was your energy like? _____

3. Notice any connections between food and mood? Between food and energy? Between food and feelings? _____

4. Any comments about what you liked or didn't like about your day? Did you come up against any obstacles today? What were they? *Who* were they? _____

5. Any final thoughts or feelings or things you need to say to complete the day for yourself?

   _____

   _____

   _____

6. Can you let what happened today be the way it was and be the way it was not? (Either a simple "yes" or "no" is okay.) _____

Day Three: _____

Goals for Today

_____

_____

_____

Food Record

_____

_____

_____

_____

_____

_____

_____

_____

_____

Exercise Today

_____

_____

_____

_____

_____

_____

_____

_____

_____

Which "A" list food was added to today's menu?

_____

End-of-the-Day Questions

1. What kind of day did you have? _____

2. What was your energy like? _____

3. Notice any connections between food and mood? Between food and energy? Between food and feelings? _____

4. Any comments about what you liked or didn't like about your day? Did you come up against any obstacles today? What were they? *Who* were they? _____
_____

5. Any final thoughts or feelings or things you need to say to complete the day for yourself?
_____
_____
_____

6. Can you let what happened today be the way it was and be the way it was not? (Either a simple "yes" or "no" is okay.) _____

Day Four: _____

Goals for Today

_____
_____
_____

Food Record

_____
_____
_____
_____
_____
_____
_____
_____
_____
_____

Exercise Today

_____
_____
_____
_____
_____
_____
_____
_____
_____

Which "A" list food was added to today's menu?

_____

End-of-the-Day Questions

1. What kind of day did you have? _____
2. What was your energy like? _____
3. Notice any connections between food and mood? Between food and energy? Between food and feelings? _____
4. Any comments about what you liked or didn't like about your day? Did you come up against any obstacles today? What were they? *Who* were they? _____
   _____
5. Any final thoughts or feelings or things you need to say to complete the day for yourself?
   _____
   _____
   _____
6. Can you let what happened today be the way it was and be the way it was not? (Either a simple "yes" or "no" is okay.) _____

Day Five: _____

Goals for Today

_____

_____

_____

Food Record

_____

_____

_____

_____

_____

_____

_____

_____

_____

Exercise Today

_____

_____

_____

_____

_____

_____

_____

_____

_____

_____

Which "A" list food was added to today's menu?

_____

End-of-the-Day Questions

1. What kind of day did you have? _____
2. What was your energy like? _____
3. Notice any connections between food and mood? Between food and energy? Between food and feelings? _____
4. Any comments about what you liked or didn't like about your day? Did you come up against any obstacles today? What were they? *Who* were they? _____
5. Any final thoughts or feelings or things you need to say to complete the day for yourself?

_____

_____

_____

6. Can you let what happened today be the way it was and be the way it was not? (Either a simple "yes" or "no" is okay.) _____

Day Six: _____

Goals for Today

_____

_____

_____

Food Record

_____

_____

_____

_____

_____

_____

_____

_____

_____

Exercise Today

_____

_____

_____

_____

_____

_____

_____

_____

_____

Which "A" list food was added to today's menu?

_____

End-of-the-Day Questions

1. What kind of day did you have? _____

2. What was your energy like? _____

3. Notice any connections between food and mood? Between food and energy? Between food and feelings? _____

4. Any comments about what you liked or didn't like about your day? Did you come up against any obstacles today? What were they? *Who* were they? _____

5. Any final thoughts or feelings or things you need to say to complete the day for yourself?

_____

_____

_____

6. Can you let what happened today be the way it was and be the way it was not? (Either a simple "yes" or "no" is okay.) _____

Day Seven: _____

Goals for Today

_____

_____

_____

Food Record

_____

_____

_____

_____

_____

_____

_____

_____

_____

Exercise Today

_____

_____

_____

_____

_____

_____

_____

_____

_____

Which "A" list food was added to today's menu?

_____

End-of-the-Day Questions

1. What kind of day did you have? _____
2. What was your energy like? _____
3. Notice any connections between food and mood? Between food and energy? Between food and feelings? _____
4. Any comments about what you liked or didn't like about your day? Did you come up against any obstacles today? What were they? *Who* were they? _____
_____
5. Any final thoughts or feelings or things you need to say to complete the day for yourself?
_____
_____
_____
6. Can you let what happened today be the way it was and be the way it was not? (Either a simple "yes" or "no" is okay.) _____

Week One Self-Evaluation Questions

Note: You can write in this section at any time during the week. If it helps you to break these questions down into categories like health, family, and work, by all means do so, but it's not necessary. Answer in any way that's comfortable for you. You might also want to break it down into long-range and short-range goals, but that's also optional.

What are your primary goals in life?

_____

_____

_____

_____

_____

_____

_____

Where would you like to be, personally and professionally, in five years?

_____

_____

_____

_____

_____

_____

How about in ten?

_____

_____

_____

_____

_____

_____

Week One Round-Up

Note: You can write in this section at any time during the week.

What are you noticing, if anything, from keeping the food journal?

_____

_____

_____

_____

What items came off your to-do list this week?

_____

_____

_____

_____

_____

_____

How are you feeling about doing the program? (Remember, feelings are not facts. You may feel terrific about it, you may hate it. You may feel both! Or you may feel anything in between. It's all okay. Just tell the truth about it.)

_____

_____

_____

_____

_____

Anything else you need to say before moving into week two?

_____

_____

_____

_____

_____

_____

WEEK TWO

WEEK TWO

A problem is a chance to do your best.

—Duke Ellington

Thirty years ago my older brother, who was ten years old at the time, was trying to get a report on birds written that he'd had three months to write. It was due the next day. We were out at our family cabin in Bolinas, and he was at the kitchen table close to tears, surrounded by binder paper and pencils and unopened books on birds, immobilized by the hugeness of the task ahead.

Then my father sat down beside him, put his arm around my brother's shoulder, and said:

"Bird by bird, buddy. Just take it bird by bird."

—Ann Lamott

The Top Ten Subversive Nutrition Facts You Need to Know About

1. *The food pyramid is not for everyone.* The idea that we need six to eleven daily servings of grains, breads, and cereals is patent nonsense for most people. For many people the overconsumption of these foods leads to bloat, fat, and ill health.

2. *There is no perfect diet.* Some people do fabulously well on vegetarian diets and some people crash and burn. One size only fits people who come in that size.

3. *All lower-carb diets are not "the Atkins Diet."* There are many ways to get the healthful, weight-reducing benefits of a lower-carb diet besides the original Atkins plan.

4. *Stress can make you fat.* The stress hormone cortisol leads to carbohydrate cravings and overeating, as well as to abdominal fat.

5. *Managing insulin levels might just be your most important anti-aging strategy.* Balance this all-important hormone and you will almost always see improvement in cholesterol and blood pressure, and reduce your risk for Type II diabetes. Protein at every meal, good fats, and fewer carbohydrates can help accomplish this.

6. *There are different metabolic types.* Some of us are Jaguars and some of us are SUVs . . . you need to match the right kind of gas (food) with the right kind of engine (metabolism).

7. *The idea that a balanced diet will provide you with everything you need is woefully out of date.* It's possible to have "minimum wage" health without supplements, but it's virtually impossible to have *optimal* health without them.

8. *Blood type can make a difference (but it's not the only thing to base a diet on).* Some blood types are far more likely to be allergic or sensitive to certain foods. Type O people, for example, are far more likely than other types to be hypersensitive to dairy foods.

9. *When it comes to heart disease, we've been way overemphasizing cholesterol.* Cholesterol is not the whole picture—it may not even be the most important part of the picture. The ratio of triglycerides to HDL, for example, is a much better predictor of heart disease than your cholesterol number.

10. *Doctors generally know no more about nutrition and supplements than you do.* The average doctor knows less about nutrition than you do. Most medical schools teach zero hours of nutrition, and in fact, subtly communicate an anti-nutritional bias.

Remember to keep writing! If you don't feel like it, jot down "I don't feel like writing today." Just stay in communication with your journal. See if you can begin to notice more connections between what you eat and how you feel. This works in both directions—how you eat may influence how you feel (your mood, energy, and self-esteem) but equally important, how you feel may influence what you eat and how much you eat. Start connecting the dots.

Food Goals

- Eliminate *one food* from the "B" list.
- Add *two foods* from the "A" list.

Exercise Goals

Beginners

- Five days a week: Walking, for ten minutes a day.
- Two days a week after walking (these are your "weight training days") do crunches

Day One	Day Two	Day Three	Day Four	Day Five
Walk 10 minutes	Walk 10 minutes Crunches	Walk 10 minutes	Walk 10 minutes Crunches	Walk 10 minutes

Intermediate/Advanced Workout

- Five days a week: Do cardio for twenty to forty minutes (walking, running, stairclimber, or stationary bike)

PLUS

- Two days a week after walking (these are your "weight training days") do crunches (two or three sets)

Day One	Day Two	Day Three	Day Four	Day Five
Cardio 20–40 min.	Cardio 20–40 min. Crunches 2–3 sets	Cardio 20–40 min.	Cardio 20–40 min. Crunches 2–3 sets	Cardio 20–40 min.

OR

- Three days a week: Cardio for twenty to forty minutes (walking, running, stairclimber, or stationary bike)

PLUS

- One day: Intermediate Workout "A" (home or gym)
- One day: Intermediate Workout "B" (home or gym)

Day One	Day Two	Day Three	Day Four	Day Five
Cardio 20–40 min.	Intermediate workout A	Cardio 20–40 min.	Intermediate workout B	Cardio 20–40 min.

To-Do List Goals

- Do at least *two more things* each day from the master to-do list. Since you're adding stuff to it all the time, you shouldn't be running out of things to do.

Day One: _____

Goals for Today

_____
_____
_____

Exercise Today

_____
_____
_____
_____
_____
_____
_____
_____
_____

Food Record

_____
_____
_____
_____
_____
_____
_____
_____
_____

Which "A" list food was added to today's menu?

_____

Which "B" list foods did you not eat?

_____

End-of-the-Day Questions

1. What kind of day did you have? _____
2. What was your energy like? _____
3. Notice any connections between food and mood? Between food and energy? Between food and feelings? _____
4. Any comments about what you liked or didn't like about your day? Did you come up against any obstacles today? What were they? *Who* were they? _____
_____
5. Any final thoughts or feelings or things you need to say to complete the day for yourself?
_____
_____
_____
6. Can you let what happened today be the way it was and be the way it was not? (Either a simple "yes" or "no" is okay.) _____

Day Two: _____

Goals for Today

_____

_____

_____

Exercise Today

_____

_____

_____

_____

_____

_____

_____

_____

_____

Food Record

_____

_____

_____

_____

_____

_____

_____

_____

_____

Which "A" list food was added to today's menu?

_____

Which "B" list foods did you not eat?

_____

End-of-the-Day Questions

1. What kind of day did you have? _____

2. What was your energy like? _____

3. Notice any connections between food and mood? Between food and energy? Between food and feelings? _____

4. Any comments about what you liked or didn't like about your day? Did you come up against any obstacles today? What were they? *Who* were they? _____

_____

5. Any final thoughts or feelings or things you need to say to complete the day for yourself?

_____

_____

_____

6. Can you let what happened today be the way it was and be the way it was not? (Either a simple "yes" or "no" is okay.) _____

Day Three: _____

Goals for Today

_____

_____

_____

Food Record

_____

_____

_____

_____

_____

_____

_____

_____

_____

Exercise Today

_____

_____

_____

_____

_____

_____

_____

_____

_____

Which "A" list food was added to today's menu?

_____

Which "B" list foods did you not eat?

_____

End-of-the-Day Questions

1. What kind of day did you have? _____

2. What was your energy like? _____

3. Notice any connections between food and mood? Between food and energy? Between food and feelings? _____

4. Any comments about what you liked or didn't like about your day? Did you come up against any obstacles today? What were they? *Who* were they? _____

_____

5. Any final thoughts or feelings or things you need to say to complete the day for yourself?

_____

_____

_____

6. Can you let what happened today be the way it was and be the way it was not? (Either a simple "yes" or "no" is okay.) _____

Day Four: _____

Goals for Today

_____

_____

_____

Food Record

_____

_____

_____

_____

_____

_____

_____

_____

_____

Exercise Today

_____

_____

_____

_____

_____

_____

_____

_____

Which "A" list food was added to today's menu?

_____

Which "B" list foods did you not eat?

_____

End-of-the-Day Questions

1. What kind of day did you have? _____
2. What was your energy like? _____
3. Notice any connections between food and mood? Between food and energy? Between food and feelings? _____
4. Any comments about what you liked or didn't like about your day? Did you come up against any obstacles today? What were they? *Who* were they? _____
   _____
5. Any final thoughts or feelings or things you need to say to complete the day for yourself?
   _____
   _____
   _____
6. Can you let what happened today be the way it was and be the way it was not? (Either a simple "yes" or "no" is okay.) _____

Day Five: _____

Goals for Today

_____
_____
_____

Food Record

_____
_____
_____
_____
_____
_____
_____
_____
_____

Exercise Today

_____
_____
_____
_____
_____
_____
_____
_____
_____

Which "A" list food was added to today's menu?

_____

Which "B" list foods did you not eat?

_____

End-of-the-Day Questions

1. What kind of day did you have? _____
2. What was your energy like? _____
3. Notice any connections between food and mood? Between food and energy? Between food and feelings? _____
4. Any comments about what you liked or didn't like about your day? Did you come up against any obstacles today? What were they? *Who* were they? _____
5. Any final thoughts or feelings or things you need to say to complete the day for yourself?
_____
_____
_____
6. Can you let what happened today be the way it was and be the way it was not? (Either a simple "yes" or "no" is okay.) _____

Day Six: _____

Goals for Today

_____

_____

_____

Food Record

_____

_____

_____

_____

_____

_____

_____

_____

_____

Exercise Today

_____

_____

_____

_____

_____

_____

_____

_____

_____

Which "A" list food was added to today's menu?

_____

Which "B" list foods did you not eat?

_____

End-of-the-Day Questions

1. What kind of day did you have? _____
2. What was your energy like? _____
3. Notice any connections between food and mood? Between food and energy? Between food and feelings? _____
4. Any comments about what you liked or didn't like about your day? Did you come up against any obstacles today? What were they? *Who* were they? _____
_____
5. Any final thoughts or feelings or things you need to say to complete the day for yourself?
_____
_____
_____
6. Can you let what happened today be the way it was and be the way it was not? (Either a simple "yes" or "no" is okay.) _____

Day Seven: _____

Goals for Today

_____
_____
_____

Food Record

_____
_____
_____
_____
_____
_____
_____
_____
_____

Exercise Today

_____
_____
_____
_____
_____
_____
_____
_____
_____

Which "A" list food was added to today's menu?

_____

Which "B" list foods did you not eat?

_____

End-of-the-Day Questions

1. What kind of day did you have? _____
2. What was your energy like? _____
3. Notice any connections between food and mood? Between food and energy? Between food and feelings? _____
4. Any comments about what you liked or didn't like about your day? Did you come up against any obstacles today? What were they? *Who* were they? _____
_____
5. Any final thoughts or feelings or things you need to say to complete the day for yourself?
_____
_____
_____
6. Can you let what happened today be the way it was and be the way it was not? (Either a simple "yes" or "no" is okay.) _____

Week Two Self-Evaluation Questions

Note: You can write in this section at any time during the week.

How would you rate your overall level of satisfaction in your day-to-day life?

_____

_____

_____

_____

_____

_____

What actions could you take right now to increase the level of personal satisfaction in your day-to-day life?

_____

_____

_____

_____

_____

_____

What obstacles, if any, do you see in taking those actions? What's standing in the way of you doing at least one of the actions you listed above *today?*

_____

_____

_____

_____

_____

Who could support you most in taking those actions? Who could you count on?

_____

_____

_____

_____

Who would *not* support you in taking those actions? Why?

_____

_____

_____

_____

_____

Week Two Round-Up

Note: You can write in this section at any time during the week.

What are you noticing, if anything, from keeping the food journal?

_____

_____

_____

_____

What items came off your to-do list this week?

_____

_____

_____

_____

_____

How are you feeling about doing the program? (Remember, feelings are not facts. You may feel terrific about it, you may hate it. You may feel both! Or you may feel anything in between. It's all okay. Just tell the truth about it.)

_____

_____

_____

_____

_____

Anything else you need to say before moving into week three?

_____

_____

_____

_____

_____

_____

_____

_____

_____

_____

_____

_____

WEIGHT AND . . . FALSE FAT

"False fat" is a term coined by Dr. Elson Haas to refer to the bloating, edema, and water retention that is often a result of eating too much of the wrong kinds of food, foods to which your particular body is sensitive. This "false fat" can easily add an extra ten pounds or more of weight—not only that, but eating these foods can contribute to creating "real" fat as well. Don't count on conventional allergists to help you figure out the foods to which you have this reaction. These reactions are allergylike responses, but they don't come under the heading of classic food allergies. Conventional allergists define "allergy" in a very specific way, as a very specific response, like, for example, a rash. But there are lots of ways your body can scream, "I don't like this food and don't know how to handle it." "Food reactions" is a better description of the phenomena than "food allergies," but the overall result is something that you don't want: both "*false* fat" and *real* fat.

Just like hay fever causes swelling in the nasal tissues and eyes, food sensitivities cause "swelling" by sending water to surround food particles that your digestive system is unable to break down properly. This is just a normal part of the inflammatory response—the body sees these "undigested" particles as foreign invaders and tries to get rid of them. One result of this is abdominal bloating and water retention.

Another is the release of stress hormones. What is one of the standard "emergency room" techniques for a major food allergy reaction? A shot of adrenaline! Why? Because this stress hormone has important anti-inflammatory properties. That's why your doctor often gives you cortizone when you have an injury. When you eat reactive foods, your body *also* puts out adrenaline and other stress hormones, as part of its own natural "emergency room response." These stress hormones make you feel better at first, but when you "crash" from the adrenaline high, you reach for more of the craved foods and the cycle begins again. To make it worse, the very foods that you crave are the ones that destabilize blood sugar, raise and lower insulin levels, and wind up putting on real fat.

It gets worse: You can easily become "addicted" to the very foods that cause this reaction. Here's how it works: The response to a "reactive" food also includes the release of the body's own opiates. As Dr. Haas points out, the presence of the reactive food in your system prevents discomfort, just as the presence of alcohol prevents discomfort in the alcoholic. Remove the reactive food and bingo: discomfort begins. Result: cravings, anxiety, and a kind of "withdrawl." Since food cravings are one of the primary reasons diet strategies fail, preventing cravings is a critically important part of any weight-loss program. And the foods that you crave are almost always the very foods that contribute to the problem of overweight in the first place!

Serotonin levels are also depressed when you eat reactive foods because serotonin is mostly carried by white blood cells, which are the very same cells used by the immune system in producing a "counterresponse" to reactive foods. Although those white blood cells are busy responding to the reactive food, they're less able to deliver serotonin to your brain. Low serotonin levels are consistently associated with cravings, depression, and the lack of a sense of well-being. Since sugar and high-carb junk foods raise serotonin levels, those are exactly the ones you tend to crave when you're in "low serotonin mode," and from a weight loss (and health) perspective they are also the ones that do the most damage.

Since many of the foods we are "reactive" to are all around us, and many of the usual suspects—like wheat—are in virtually everything, detoxification and rotation diets are often a good idea. If you're stuck on a plateau or are experiencing any of the symptoms discussed like fatigue, bloat, or "brain fog," try removing what Dr. Haas calls "the seven most reactive foods: dairy, wheat, corn, sugar, soy, eggs, and peanuts." At the very least, try taking out dairy, wheat, and sugar (all "B" and "C" list foods) and see how you feel. The Shape-Up friendly "A" list has virtually none of the "usual suspects" for food sensitivities.

Resource: *The False Fat Diet* by Dr. Elson Haas

The Top Ten Ways to Jump-Start Weight Loss

1. Eat protein at every meal, including breakfast.
2. Eliminate wheat- and flour-based products for the time being. And yes, that definitely includes bread and pasta.
3. Eliminate "food products." Ninety percent of what you eat should be food that could have been hunted, caught, gathered from the ground, plucked from a tree, or grown.
4. Reduce starch. When you do eat starches, choose from "real" carbohydrates. The best choices are oatmeal, sweet potatoes, beans, and legumes.
5. Don't eat unlimited amounts of fruit and be careful with the extra-sweet, extra-ripe variety. For now, keep fruits to two a day, and choose the low-sugar, high-fiber variety. Apples, pears, plums, and especially berries all are good choices. For now, fruit should be eaten alone or with something light like nuts or a little cheese. Lose the fruit juice.
6. Reduce or eliminate dairy foods for the time being, especially cow's milk. Exceptions: reasonable amounts of cheese and occasional portions of yogurt, but not the fat-free kind (it contains way too much sugar).
7. Try eliminating alcohol. You can always go back to moderate drinking later on if it works for you.

8. Stop using vegetable oils such as sunflower, safflower, and corn. Vegetable oils in the supermarket are highly refined and oxidize easily when heated, contributing to arterial plaque.

9. Worry less about the *amount* of fat you eat and pay more attention to the *kind* of fat you eat. The worst kinds of fat are in fried foods, margarine, and foods that contain hydrogenated or partially hydrogenated oils. The best are the omega-3's, found in fish and flaxseed oil.

10. Drink at least eight or more large glasses of pure water a day. Every day. No excuses.

WEEK THREE

WEEK THREE

If you strive for thin you'll never win.

Strive for health and thin will follow.

—ELSON HAAS, M.D.

Whatever you do, keep writing. What have you noticed in the last two weeks? Have there been any obvious connections between food and mood? How about not-so-obvious connections? What's your energy been like? Have you noticed any resentment about doing these processes? A sense of elation? Empowerment? Discouragement? Sadness? Hopefulness? Hope*less*ness? All of the above? None of the above? Write it down! And here's one further assignment for the week: Be willing to be wherever you are with this. As you'll discover as you do this program, despite our best efforts to the contrary, the only place we can be is where we are. Whatever you're going through, be with it. Just keep telling the truth about it, and keep looking.

And when you think there's nothing more to do . . .

Look some more.

Food Goals

- Add one more food from the "A" list.
- Eliminate one more food from the "B" list.
- Have protein at each meal. You don't have to weigh and measure, but if you're comfortable with doing so, roughly three or four ounces equals one serving of protein—but don't lose any sleep over being exact at this point. A serving generally fits into a medium-size hand.

Exercise Goals

Beginners

- Five days a week: Walking, for twenty minutes a day
- Two days a week after walking (these are your "weight training days"): crunches and squats

Day One	Day Two	Day Three	Day Four	Day Five
Walk 20 min.	Walk 20 min. Crunches Squats	Walk 20 min.	Walk 20 min. Crunches Squats	Walk 20 min.

Intermediate/Advanced Workout

- Five days a week: Cardio for thirty to forty minutes (walking, running, stair-climber, or stationary bike)
PLUS
- Two days a week after walking (these are your "weight training days"): crunches (two to three sets), squats (two to three sets)

Day One	Day Two	Day Three	Day Four	Day Five
Cardio 30–40 min.	Cardio 30–40 min. Crunches 2–3 sets Squats 2–3 sets	Cardio 30–40 min.	Cardio 30–40 min. Crunches 2–3 sets Squats 2–3 sets	Cardio 30–40 min

OR

- Three days a week: Cardio for thirty to forty minutes (walking, running, stair-climber, or stationary bike)

PLUS

- One day: Intermediate Workout "A" (home or gym)
- One day: Intermediate Workout "B" (home or gym)

Day One	Day Two	Day Three	Day Four	Day Five
Cardio 30–40 min.	Intermediate workout A	Cardio 30–40 min.	Intermediate workout B	Cardio 30–40 min

To-Do List Goals

- Expand the list and add any new items you think of that feel like they belong on the list.
- Do at least two tasks from the master to-do list per day. Any two. Check them off when you complete them, and enter them in the Week Three Round-Up.

Hint: No item is too "insignificant." It all counts.

Day One: _____

Goals for Today

_____
_____
_____

Food Record

_____
_____
_____
_____
_____
_____
_____
_____

Exercise Today

_____
_____
_____
_____
_____
_____
_____
_____

Which "A" list food was added to today's menu?

_____

Which "B" list foods did you not eat?

_____

Protein at each meal?

_____

End-of-the-Day Questions

1. What kind of day did you have? _____
2. What was your energy like? _____
3. Notice any connections between food and mood? Between food and energy? Between food and feelings? _____
4. Any comments about what you liked or didn't like about your day? Did you come up against any obstacles today? What were they? *Who* were they? _____
_____
5. Any final thoughts or feelings or things you need to say to complete the day for yourself?
_____
_____
_____
6. Can you let what happened today be the way it was and be the way it was not? (Either a simple "yes" or "no" is okay.) _____

Day Two: _____

Goals for Today

_____
_____
_____

Food Record

_____
_____
_____
_____
_____
_____
_____
_____
_____

Exercise Today

_____
_____
_____
_____
_____
_____
_____
_____

Which "A" list food was added to today's menu?

_____

Which "B" list foods did you not eat?

_____

Protein at each meal?

_____

End-of-the-Day Questions

1. What kind of day did you have? _____
2. What was your energy like? _____
3. Notice any connections between food and mood? Between food and energy? Between food and feelings? _____
4. Any comments about what you liked or didn't like about your day? Did you come up against any obstacles today? What were they? *Who* were they? _____
   _____
5. Any final thoughts or feelings or things you need to say to complete the day for yourself?
   _____
   _____
   _____
6. Can you let what happened today be the way it was and be the way it was not? (Either a simple "yes" or "no" is okay.) _____

Day Three: _____

Goals for Today

_____

_____

_____

Food Record

_____

_____

_____

_____

_____

_____

_____

_____

Exercise Today

_____

_____

_____

_____

_____

_____

_____

_____

Which "A" list food was added to today's menu?

_____

Which "B" list foods did you not eat?

_____

Protein at each meal?

_____

End-of-the-Day Questions

1. What kind of day did you have? _____
2. What was your energy like? _____
3. Notice any connections between food and mood? Between food and energy? Between food and feelings? _____
4. Any comments about what you liked or didn't like about your day? Did you come up against any obstacles today? What were they? *Who* were they? _____
5. Any final thoughts or feelings or things you need to say to complete the day for yourself?

   _____

   _____

   _____

6. Can you let what happened today be the way it was and be the way it was not? (Either a simple "yes" or "no" is okay.) _____

Day Four: _____

Goals for Today

_____
_____
_____

Exercise Today

_____
_____
_____
_____
_____
_____
_____
_____

Food Record

_____
_____
_____
_____
_____
_____
_____
_____
_____

Which "A" list food was added to today's menu?

_____

Which "B" list foods did you not eat?

_____

Protein at each meal?

_____

End-of-the-Day Questions

1. What kind of day did you have? _____
2. What was your energy like? _____
3. Notice any connections between food and mood? Between food and energy? Between food and feelings? _____
4. Any comments about what you liked or didn't like about your day? Did you come up against any obstacles today? What were they? *Who* were they? _____
_____
5. Any final thoughts or feelings or things you need to say to complete the day for yourself?
_____
_____
_____
6. Can you let what happened today be the way it was and be the way it was not? (Either a simple "yes" or "no" is okay.) _____

Day Five: _____

Goals for Today

_____
_____
_____

Food Record

_____
_____
_____
_____
_____
_____
_____
_____

Exercise Today

_____
_____
_____
_____
_____
_____
_____
_____

Which "A" list food was added to today's menu?

_____

Which "B" list foods did you not eat?

_____

Protein at each meal?

_____

End-of-the-Day Questions

1. What kind of day did you have? _____
2. What was your energy like? _____
3. Notice any connections between food and mood? Between food and energy? Between food and feelings? _____
4. Any comments about what you liked or didn't like about your day? Did you come up against any obstacles today? What were they? *Who* were they? _____
5. Any final thoughts or feelings or things you need to say to complete the day for yourself?
_____
_____
_____
6. Can you let what happened today be the way it was and be the way it was not? (Either a simple "yes" or "no" is okay.) _____

Day Six: _____

Goals for Today

_____
_____
_____

Food Record

_____
_____
_____
_____
_____
_____
_____
_____

Exercise Today

_____
_____
_____
_____
_____
_____
_____
_____

Which "A" list food was added to today's menu?

_____

Which "B" list foods did you not eat?

_____

Protein at each meal?

_____

End-of-the-Day Questions

1. What kind of day did you have? _____
2. What was your energy like? _____
3. Notice any connections between food and mood? Between food and energy? Between food and feelings? _____
4. Any comments about what you liked or didn't like about your day? Did you come up against any obstacles today? What were they? *Who* were they? _____
   _____
5. Any final thoughts or feelings or things you need to say to complete the day for yourself?
   _____
   _____
   _____
6. Can you let what happened today be the way it was and be the way it was not? (Either a simple "yes" or "no" is okay.) _____

Day Seven: _____

Goals for Today

_____

_____

_____

Exercise Today

_____

_____

_____

_____

_____

_____

_____

_____

Food Record

_____

_____

_____

_____

_____

_____

_____

_____

_____

Which "A" list food was added to today's menu?

_____

Which "B" list foods did you not eat?

_____

Protein at each meal?

_____

End-of-the-Day Questions

1. What kind of day did you have? _____
2. What was your energy like? _____
3. Notice any connections between food and mood? Between food and energy? Between food and feelings? _____
4. Any comments about what you liked or didn't like about your day? Did you come up against any obstacles today? What were they? *Who* were they? _____
   _____
5. Any final thoughts or feelings or things you need to say to complete the day for yourself?
   _____
   _____
   _____
6. Can you let what happened today be the way it was and be the way it was not? (Either a simple "yes" or "no" is okay.) _____

Week Three Self-Evaluation Questions

Note: You can write in this section at any time during the week

On a day-to-day basis how much thought do you give to your health and well-being? What do you think of when you think of the words "health" and "well-being"? What do they mean to you?

_____

_____

_____

_____

_____

_____

_____

How do you foresee your health and well-being ten years from now?

_____

_____

_____

_____

_____

_____

Week Three Round-Up

Note: You can write in this section at any time during the week

What are you noticing, if anything, from keeping the food journal?

_____

_____

_____

_____

What items came off your to-do list this week?

_____

_____

_____

_____

How are you feeling about doing the program? (Remember, feelings are not facts. You may feel terrific about it, you may hate it. You may feel both! Or you may feel anything in between. It's all okay. Just tell the truth about it.)

_____

_____

_____

_____

_____

Anything else you need to say before moving into week four?

_____

_____

_____

_____

_____

_____

_____

_____

_____

_____

_____

_____

_____

_____

_____

_____

WEIGHT AND . . . CRAVINGS

What you crave may also tell you a lot about the cause of the craving. According to both Julia Ross, author of *The Diet Cure,* and Kathleen Des Maisons, author of *Potatoes Not Prozac,* craving mostly sugary foods may well be linked to low levels of serotonin and endorphins. If this sounds like you, a diet higher in protein and good quality fats may help. Refined flours, sugar, and alcohol play havoc with your blood sugar and set you up for cravings, whereas protein, fat, and fiber will tend to keep blood sugar steadier and help keep cravings at bay. If you crave mostly fatty foods, your body may be telling you that you are low in essential fatty acids. Try eating more fish or supplementing with fish oil, flaxseed oil, or both. If you choose the supplement route, make sure you are also taking a multiple vitamin with minerals high in antioxidants such as vitamins E and C and selenium. Some cravings for food are actually thirst in disguise. Since most of us walk around underhydrated, half the time what we perceive as hunger is really thirst. You can test that by drinking a couple of glasses of water, preferably with a slice of lemon, waiting a few minutes, and noticing if you're still hungry. You may be surprised to see that much of the craving has disappeared.

Have you ever noticed that foods that seem irresistible at night—like dessert after dinner—don't seem very appealing at eight in the morning? That, to me, seems like a good argument that it's not the food itself that's calling you, it's your own fluctuations in blood sugar, insulin, and stress levels that have taken place during the day that make you susceptible to the food's siren song by the time evening comes around. Once again, a diet higher in protein, good quality fats, vegetables and the occasional fruit, and lower in processed, manufactured junk like commercial cereals, breads, and pastas can go a long way toward smoothing out those blood sugar roller coasters that feed the need for sweets later in the day.

Incidentally, the supplement L-glutamine, an amino acid usually available in powder form, is miraculous for curbing sweet cravings. A spoonful in some water will usually do it. Also worth trying is the herb gymnema, also known as gymnema sylvestre.

Though many people recommend dealing with cravings by having "just a little" of the food you crave, this is not always a great idea. Although it may work for some people, for sugar sensitive folks it sets up a cascade of bio-chemical processes that invariably translates to an overwhelming desire— "gimme more!" For people who are really sugar sensitive, one bite of a chocolate chip cookie is like an alcoholic having one sip of wine. If this sounds like you, having "just a little" is really not a great solution. On the other hand, if you are the kind of person who can really have just a drop of the craved food and be done with it, then I say go for it. However, I haven't met many people who are battling weight and sugar addictions who can really do that. Their brain chemistries are just not set up for the kind of "moderation" that works with people who are not wired the way they are. There's certainly no disgrace in that, and there's a whole lot of power in acknowledging it.

RESOURCES

For more on the relationship between food, cravings, biochemistry, addiction, and depression, see: *Potatoes Not Prozac* by Kathleen Des Maisones, Ph.D.; *The Sugar Addict's Total Recovery Program* by Kathleeen Des Maisones, Ph.D.; *The Diet Cure* by Julia Ross, M.A.; and *Depression Free Naturally: 7 Weeks to Eliminating Anxiety, Despair, Fatigue and Anger from Your Life* by Joan Mathews Larson, Ph.D.

The Top Ten Ways to Cut Back on Sugar

Don't add it to foods. This is the easiest and most basic way to immediately reduce the amount of sugar you're eating. Biggest targets: cereal, coffee, and tea.

Don't be fooled by "healthy sugar" disguises. Brown sugar, turbinado sugar, raw sugar . . . it's all pretty much the same thing as far as your body is concerned.

Make a real effort to reduce or eliminate processed carbohydrates. Most processed carbs—breads, bagels, most pastas, and snacks—are loaded with flour and other ingredients that convert to sugar in the body almost as fast as pure glucose. That sugar gets stored as triglycerides, which is a fancy way of saying fat.

Watch out for "fat-free" snacks. One of the biggest myths is that if a food is fat-free it doesn't make you fat. Fat-free doesn't mean calorie-free, and most fat-free snacks are loaded with sugar.

Shop for color. The more your grocery basket looks like a cornucopia of color, the better. It usually means you're getting more fresh vegetables and low-glycemic fruits such as berries and cherries.

Become a food detective. This tip is from the wonderful author and nutritionist Ann Louise Gittleman, who adds that "to reduce sugar, you have to know where it is first." Start reading labels.

Beware of artificial sweeteners. Unfortunately, they can increase cravings for sugar and carbohydrates. They can also deplete the body's stores of chromium, a nutrient crucial for blood-sugar metabolism.

Do the math. Look at the label where it says "total sugars" and divide the number of grams by four. That's the number of teaspoons of sugar you are ingesting and that's just "per serving." Want a laugh? Read the "serving size"—most "servings" have nothing to do with what normal people eat. This exercise alone should scare the pants off you.

Limit fruit (notice I didn't say "eliminate") and add more vegetables. Fruit has sugar, but it also has fiber and good nutrients. Just don't overdo it. For weight-loss purposes, two servings a day, and try to make most of them low-glycemic (see p. 49).

Eliminate fruit juice. It's a pure sugar hit with none of the fiber and less of the nutrients that are found in the fruit itself.

WEEK FOUR

It is our choices that show what we truly are, far more than our abilities.

—J. K. ROWLING, HARRY POTTER AND THE CHAMBER OF SECRETS

Continue to record feelings, thoughts, impressions, mood, food, and exercise in your journal. Just stay in communication with it. Notice what your mind puts you through over this one. Maybe you don't feel like writing—what do you think about having that thought? Does it take you on a journey like "maybe this whole thing is useless," "I'll never be able to do it," "the assignments are stupid," "I'm sure I'm not doing it right"? Does it take you on a different journey? Does it take you *out* of the journey? Remember, wherever you're going with this, you're living in your head if you're engaging in this chatter. It's useless chatter, except insofar as it teaches you something about what it's like to live in your head! Chatter all you want—just stay in communication with the journal!

Food Goals

- Add one more food from the "A" list (more if you want to).
- Eliminate one more food from the "B" list.

Exercise Goals

Beginners

- Five days a week: Walking, for thirty minutes a day
- Two days a week after walking (these are your "weight training days"): crunches, squats, chest presses, and one-arm rows

Day One	Day Two	Day Three	Day Four	Day Five
Walk 30 min.	Walk 30 min. Crunches Squats Chest presses One-arm rows	Walk 30 min.	Walk 30 min. Crunches Squats Chest presses One-arm rows	Walk 30 min.

Intermediate/Advanced Workout

- Five days a week: Cardio for thirty to forty minutes (walking, running, stair-climber, or stationary bike)*

  *(optional: try adding speed intervals of thirty to ninety seconds mixed in)

PLUS

- Two days a week after walking (these are your "weight training days"): crunches (two to three sets), squats (two to three sets), chest presses (two to three sets), one-arm rows (two to three sets)

Day One	Day Two	Day Three	Day Four	Day Five
Cardio 30–40 min.	Cardio 30–40 min. Crunches 2–3 sets Squats 2–3 sets Chest presses 2–3 sets One-arm rows 2–3 sets	Cardio 30–40 min.	Cardio 30–40 min. Crunches 2–3 sets Squats 2–3 sets Chest presses 2–3 sets One-arm rows 2–3 sets	Cardio 30–40 min.

OR

- Three days a week: Cardio for twenty to forty minutes (walking, running, stairclimber, or stationary bike)

PLUS

- One day: Intermediate Workout "A" (home or gym)
- One day: Intermediate Workout "B" (home or gym)

Day One	Day Two	Day Three	Day Four	Day Five
Cardio 20–40 min.	Intermediate workout A	Cardio 20–40 min.	Intermediate workout B	Cardio 20–40 min.

To-Do List Goals

- Complete at least two more tasks on the list.

Day One: _____

Goals for Today

_____

_____

_____

Food Record

_____

_____

_____

_____

_____

_____

_____

_____

Exercise Today

_____

_____

_____

_____

_____

_____

_____

_____

Which "A" list food was added to today's menu?

_____

Which "B" list foods did you not eat?

_____

Protein at each meal?

_____

End-of-the-Day Questions

1. What kind of day did you have? _____

2. What was your energy like? _____

3. Notice any connections between food and mood? Between food and energy? Between food and feelings? _____

4. Any comments about what you liked or didn't like about your day? Did you come up against any obstacles today? What were they? *Who* were they? _____

5. Any final thoughts or feelings or things you need to say to complete the day for yourself?

_____

_____

_____

6. Can you let what happened today be the way it was and be the way it was not? (Either a simple "yes" or "no" is okay.) _____

Day Two: _____

Goals for Today

_____
_____
_____

Food Record

_____
_____
_____
_____
_____
_____
_____
_____

Exercise Today

_____
_____
_____
_____
_____
_____
_____
_____

Which "A" list food was added to today's menu?

_____

Which "B" list foods did you not eat?

_____

Protein at each meal?

_____

End-of-the-Day Questions

1. What kind of day did you have? _____
2. What was your energy like? _____
3. Notice any connections between food and mood? Between food and energy? Between food and feelings? _____
4. Any comments about what you liked or didn't like about your day? Did you come up against any obstacles today? What were they? *Who* were they? _____
5. Any final thoughts or feelings or things you need to say to complete the day for yourself?
_____
_____
_____
6. Can you let what happened today be the way it was and be the way it was not? (Either a simple "yes" or "no" is okay.) _____

Day Three: _____

Goals for Today

_____

_____

_____

Food Record

_____

_____

_____

_____

_____

_____

_____

_____

Exercise Today

_____

_____

_____

_____

_____

_____

_____

_____

Which "A" list food was added to today's menu?

_____

Which "B" list foods did you not eat?

_____

Protein at each meal?

_____

End-of-the-Day Questions

1. What kind of day did you have? _____
2. What was your energy like? _____
3. Notice any connections between food and mood? Between food and energy? Between food and feelings? _____
4. Any comments about what you liked or didn't like about your day? Did you come up against any obstacles today? What were they? *Who* were they? _____
   _____
5. Any final thoughts or feelings or things you need to say to complete the day for yourself?
   _____
   _____
   _____
6. Can you let what happened today be the way it was and be the way it was not? (Either a simple "yes" or "no" is okay.) _____

Day Four: _____

Goals for Today

_____
_____
_____

Food Record

_____
_____
_____
_____
_____
_____
_____
_____

Exercise Today

_____
_____
_____
_____
_____
_____
_____
_____

Which "A" list food was added to today's menu?

_____

Which "B" list foods did you not eat?

_____

Protein at each meal?

_____

End-of-the-Day Questions

1. What kind of day did you have? _____
2. What was your energy like? _____
3. Notice any connections between food and mood? Between food and energy? Between food and feelings? _____
4. Any comments about what you liked or didn't like about your day? Did you come up against any obstacles today? What were they? *Who* were they? _____

5. Any final thoughts or feelings or things you need to say to complete the day for yourself?
_____
_____
_____

6. Can you let what happened today be the way it was and be the way it was not? (Either a simple "yes" or "no" is okay.) _____

Day Five: _____

Goals for Today

_____

_____

_____

Food Record

_____

_____

_____

_____

_____

_____

_____

_____

_____

Exercise Today

_____

_____

_____

_____

_____

_____

_____

Which "A" list food was added to today's menu?

_____

Which "B" list foods did you not eat?

_____

Protein at each meal?

_____

End-of-the-Day Questions

1. What kind of day did you have? _____
2. What was your energy like? _____
3. Notice any connections between food and mood? Between food and energy? Between food and feelings? _____
4. Any comments about what you liked or didn't like about your day? Did you come up against any obstacles today? What were they? *Who* were they? _____
   _____
5. Any final thoughts or feelings or things you need to say to complete the day for yourself?
   _____
   _____
   _____
6. Can you let what happened today be the way it was and be the way it was not? (Either a simple "yes" or "no" is okay.) _____

Day Six: _____

Goals for Today

_____
_____
_____

Food Record

_____
_____
_____
_____
_____
_____
_____
_____
_____

Exercise Today

_____
_____
_____
_____
_____
_____
_____
_____

Which "A" list food was added to today's menu?

_____

Which "B" list foods did you not eat?

_____

Protein at each meal?

_____

End-of-the-Day Questions

1. What kind of day did you have? _____

2. What was your energy like? _____

3. Notice any connections between food and mood? Between food and energy? Between food and feelings? _____

4. Any comments about what you liked or didn't like about your day? Did you come up against any obstacles today? What were they? *Who* were they? _____

5. Any final thoughts or feelings or things you need to say to complete the day for yourself? _____
   _____
   _____

6. Can you let what happened today be the way it was and be the way it was not? (Either a simple "yes" or "no" is okay.) _____

Day Seven: _____

Goals for Today

_____

_____

_____

Food Record

_____

_____

_____

_____

_____

_____

_____

_____

Exercise Today

_____

_____

_____

_____

_____

_____

_____

Which "A" list food was added to today's menu?

_____

Which "B" list foods did you not eat?

_____

Protein at each meal?

_____

End-of-the-Day Questions

1. What kind of day did you have? _____
2. What was your energy like? _____
3. Notice any connections between food and mood? Between food and energy? Between food and feelings? _____
4. Any comments about what you liked or didn't like about your day? Did you come up against any obstacles today? What were they? *Who* were they? _____
_____
5. Any final thoughts or feelings or things you need to say to complete the day for yourself?
_____
_____
_____
6. Can you let what happened today be the way it was and be the way it was not? (Either a simple "yes" or "no" is okay.) _____

Week Four Self-Evaluation Questions

Note: You can write in this section at any time during the week.

What, if anything, would you most like to change about your life?

_____

_____

_____

_____

_____

_____

_____

_____

How could you accomplish this?

_____

_____

_____

_____

_____

_____

_____

_____

(By the way, I just want to remind you that there is no "right" way to do these exercises or answer these questions. So if, for example, the only way you can imagine changing some aspect of your life means being whimsical or doing something outrageous, go ahead and write it down. Maybe it'll be something concrete you could do, maybe it'll be something completely fanciful. Maybe you'd like to be a contestant on a reality show. Maybe you'd like to run off with the pool boy (or girl). Maybe you'd like to have grandkids or go back to medical school. It doesn't have to be practical. It just has to be something you've thought of, even if you've just thought of it now for the first time and it doesn't make any sense. See where it takes you. Maybe nowhere. Maybe . . . who knows? Write it down!)

Week Four Round-Up

Note: You can write in this section at any time during the week.

What are you noticing, if anything, from keeping the food journal?

_____
_____
_____
_____

What items came off your to-do list this week?

_____
_____
_____
_____
_____
_____

How are you feeling about doing the program? (Remember, feelings are not facts. You may feel terrific about it, you may hate it. You may feel both! Or you may feel anything in between. It's all okay. Just tell the truth about it.)

_____
_____
_____
_____
_____

Anything else you need to say before moving into week five?

_____
_____
_____
_____
_____

WEIGHT AND . . . PMS

Hormones have a significant influence on weight gain for both sexes, but perhaps even more so for women. Estrogen has a profound effect on fat gain, both directly and indirectly. In addition, the monthly *fluctuations* of estrogen and progesterone in premenopausal women have an enormous effect on cravings and on the overall sense of well-being, both of which, in turn, have an enormous effect on eating behavior. These fluctuations remain a factor all the way through the completion of menopause.

Estrogen is a kind of "natural" antidepressant. (Anyone remember the old bumper sticker "I'm out of estrogen and I have a gun"?) Through a complicated feedback loop, estrogen affects your body's production of a compound called serotonin, a feel-good neurotransmitter that's involved in feelings of "being okay" and also in the ability to resist impulses. Low estrogen equals low serotonin. Low serotonin equals cravings, almost always for high-carbohydrate, high-sugar foods (think chocolate, for example).

Progesterone, however, also affects feelings of well-being. It's the parent hormone for stress hormones, so when you are stressed, you have even less of it. The delicate balance between these hormones—estrogen and progesterone—is critical. They have complementary and opposing effects on mood, with serotonin being a mood elevator and progesterone being a natural relaxant. Too much estrogen in relation to progesterone may also lead to weight gain and fluid retention (one possible mechanism for women on the pill experiencing weight gain). During the second (luteinizing) phase of the menstrual cycle, estrogen is lowest in relation to progesterone, and this is the time frame when mood swings and cravings are greatest, although this may be more due to the sudden *fluctuations* and imbalances between estrogen and progesterone than to the absolute levels of either hormone alone.

Serotonin is also the precursor for another important hormone called melatonin. Melatonin is made in the pineal gland and helps you to sleep. Low serotonin equals low melatonin. Most of us aren't getting anywhere near enough sleep to begin with, so anything that makes sleep more difficult—like inadequate levels of melatonin, for example—adds to stress and to the body's production of stress hormones. More stress equals more cravings, and more stress hormones mean more fat storage.

Why not just "give in" to the cravings and medicate ourselves a little with some high-carb junk foods and be done with it? On the surface this seems to make sense, but it's really not the best idea. When we "give in" to the cravings for high-sugar carbohydrates we go back on the blood sugar roller coaster, and also raise insulin levels, making fat storage a lot more likely. This can make us even more depressed, and the cycle continues. Sugar sensitive people—also known as sugar addicts or carbohydrate addicts—get into even more trouble with this strategy. When they go off on a sugar binge, even a mild one, their brain lights up as if they just hit the chemical version of *Double Jeopardy.* This sets them up for an even more intense go-round of further cravings and addictive behavior.

PMS—or low estrogen levels—are made much worse by caffeine. Caffeine stimulates the adrenals and raises levels of the stress hormone cortisol, making it far less likely that you will feel relaxed; this intensifies a "low serotonin" state in which you are very vulnerable to cravings.

Many people choose to simply medicate the low-serotonin state with drugs like Prozac, but there are other ways to affect it such as diet, stress reduction, and relationships with others. Since serotonin is made from the amino acid tryptophan, which is found in proteins such as turkey, adequate protein is a must. The body has an amazing mechanism for keeing tryptophan on hand for when it is most needed, which is at night, both for relaxing and for metabolic repair. Eat protein throughout the day and make sure to have some "real food" carbohydrates later in the day (like the ones on the "A" list) to help provide an escort for this tryptophan to get into the brain where it can transform into serotonin.

Studies have shown that PMS sufferers consume more sugar, refined carbohydrates, sodium, and dairy and less zinc, magnesium, and iron than non-PMS sufferers. The more you switch to "A" list foods, the less likely you will be to have these nutritional deficiencies and imbalances. Heads up: More and more research is now pointing to the profound affect of the fats found in fish oils on even the most difficult depressive states.

As Dr. Diana Schwarzbein puts it, the low serotonin state can be healed but you have to go through the healing process. There are also a number of ways to raise serotonin that have nothing to do with drugs or diet. Dr. Kathleen Des Maisones (author of *Potatoes not Prozac*) mentions a number of them: Good sex. Good friends. Relatedness. Being in the sun. Having a relationship with an animal. Being part of a group (a big part of why twelve-step programs work, by the way). Doing good things for other people. Every single one of these things measurably raises serotonin levels in the body and makes you feel good in the process.

Those suffering from mild PMS may also want to try the Shape-Up "PMS cocktail": 400 milligrams of magnesium, 50 milligrams of vitamin B6, and 1,000 milligrams of evening primrose oil twice a day, beginning ten days before your actual cycle. Magnesium is a "relaxing" mineral, B6 is needed to convert tryptophan into serotonin, and evening primrose oil contains an important fatty acid (GLA) that can help to balance out hormone levels. Many people have had terrific results with the combination of a Shape-Up-friendly "real food" diet and this particular supplement "cocktail."

WEEK FIVE

*Power is standing strongly in your own center
and living from your heart.*

—SARK

*Life is change.
Growth is optional.*

—KAREN KAISER CLARK

Keep writing.

Oh, and by the way . . . once in a while, when you're sure you have no more to write about, nothing more to say . . . keep writing.

Food Goals

- Now we're going to start playing a little closer attention to our carbohydrate intake. It's time to start fine tuning. If you're not noticing any changes yet, or even if you are, it's time to adjust that carbohydrate intake from the "B" list and bring it down a little further. Nothing ridiculous, mind you. Just look at it like a budget you're trying to trim. Where's the excess? Start trimming!

Exercise Goals

Beginners

- Two days a week: Walking for forty-five minutes a day
- One day a week: Walking for thirty minutes
- Two days a week: Walking for twenty minutes; then crunches, squats, chest presses, one-arm rows, bicep curls, tricep dips (these are your "weight training days")

Day One	Day Two	Day Three	Day Four	Day Five
Walk 45 min.	Walk 20 min. Crunches Squats Chest presses One-arm rows Bicep curls Tricep dips	Walk 30 min.	Walk 20 min. Crunches Squats Chest presses One-arm rows Bicep curls Tricep dips	Walk 45 min.

Intermediate/Advanced Workout

- Three days a week: Cardio for forty-five minutes (walking, running, stair-climber, or stationary bike)
- Two days a week: Cardio for twenty to thirty minutes (walking, running, stairclimber, or stationary bike); then crunches, squats, chest presses, one-arm rows, bicep curls, tricep dips, two to three sets each exercise (these are your "weight training days")

Day One	Day Two	Day Three	Day Four	Day Five
Cardio 45 min.	Cardio 20–30 min. Crunches 2–3 sets Squats 2–3 sets Chest presses 2–3 sets One-arm rows 2–3 sets Bicep curls 2–3 sets Tricep dips 2–3 sets	Cardio 45 min.	Cardio 20–30 min. Crunches 2–3 sets Squats 2–3 sets Chest presses 2–3 sets One-arm rows 2–3 sets Bicep curls 2–3 sets Tricep dips 2–3 sets	Cardio 45 min.

OR

- Three days a week: Cardio for forty-five minutes (walking, running, stair-climber, or stationary bike)

PLUS

- Two days: Intermediate Workout "C" (home or gym)
- One day: Something fun and active such as tennis, tae-bo, golf, group fitness class, yoga, hiking, playing

Day One	Day Two	Day Three	Day Four	Day Five	Day Six
Cardio 45 min.	Intermediate workout C	Cardio 45 min.	Intermediate workout C	Cardio 45 min.	Activity/fun

To-Do List Goals

- Two more things come off the list.
  Noticing anything about this? Write it down in your journal!

Day One: _____

Goals for Today

_____

_____

_____

Food Record

_____

_____

_____

_____

_____

_____

_____

_____

Exercise Today

_____

_____

_____

_____

_____

_____

_____

_____

Which "A" list food was added to today's menu?

_____

Which "B" list foods did you not eat?

_____

Protein at each meal?

_____

End-of-the-Day Questions

1. What kind of day did you have? _____
2. What was your energy like? _____
3. Notice any connections between food and mood? Between food and energy? Between food and feelings? _____
4. Any comments about what you liked or didn't like about your day? Did you come up against any obstacles today? What were they? *Who* were they? _____
   _____
5. Any final thoughts or feelings or things you need to say to complete the day for yourself?
   _____
   _____
   _____
6. Can you let what happened today be the way it was and be the way it was not? (Either a simple "yes" or "no" is okay.) _____

Day Two: _____

Goals for Today

_____
_____
_____

Food Record

_____
_____
_____
_____
_____
_____
_____
_____
_____
_____

Exercise Today

_____
_____
_____
_____
_____
_____
_____
_____

Which "A" list food was added to today's menu?

_____

Which "B" list foods did you not eat?

_____

Protein at each meal?

_____

End-of-the-Day Questions

1. What kind of day did you have? _____
2. What was your energy like? _____
3. Notice any connections between food and mood? Between food and energy? Between food and feelings? _____
4. Any comments about what you liked or didn't like about your day? Did you come up against any obstacles today? What were they? *Who* were they? _____
   _____
5. Any final thoughts or feelings or things you need to say to complete the day for yourself?
   _____
   _____
   _____
6. Can you let what happened today be the way it was and be the way it was not? (Either a simple "yes" or "no" is okay.) _____

Day Three: _____

Goals for Today

_____
_____
_____

Food Record

_____
_____
_____
_____
_____
_____
_____
_____
_____

Exercise Today

_____
_____
_____
_____
_____
_____
_____
_____

Which "A" list food was added to today's menu?

_____

Which "B" list foods did you not eat?

_____

Protein at each meal?

_____

End-of-the-Day Questions

1. What kind of day did you have? _____
2. What was your energy like? _____
3. Notice any connections between food and mood? Between food and energy? Between food and feelings? _____
4. Any comments about what you liked or didn't like about your day? Did you come up against any obstacles today? What were they? *Who* were they? _____
_____
5. Any final thoughts or feelings or things you need to say to complete the day for yourself?
_____
_____
_____
6. Can you let what happened today be the way it was and be the way it was not? (Either a simple "yes" or "no" is okay.) _____

Day Four: _____

Goals for Today

_____

_____

_____

Food Record

_____

_____

_____

_____

_____

_____

_____

_____

_____

Exercise Today

_____

_____

_____

_____

_____

_____

_____

_____

Which "A" list food was added to today's menu?

_____

Which "B" list foods did you not eat?

_____

Protein at each meal?

_____

End-of-the-Day Questions

1. What kind of day did you have? _____
2. What was your energy like? _____
3. Notice any connections between food and mood? Between food and energy? Between food and feelings? _____
4. Any comments about what you liked or didn't like about your day? Did you come up against any obstacles today? What were they? *Who* were they? _____
5. Any final thoughts or feelings or things you need to say to complete the day for yourself?

   _____

   _____

   _____

6. Can you let what happened today be the way it was and be the way it was not? (Either a simple "yes" or "no" is okay.) _____

Day Five: _____

Goals for Today

_____

_____

_____

Food Record

_____

_____

_____

_____

_____

_____

_____

_____

Exercise Today

_____

_____

_____

_____

_____

_____

_____

_____

Which "A" list food was added to today's menu?

_____

Which "B" list foods did you not eat?

_____

Protein at each meal?

_____

End-of-the-Day Questions

1. What kind of day did you have? _____
2. What was your energy like? _____
3. Notice any connections between food and mood? Between food and energy? Between food and feelings? _____
4. Any comments about what you liked or didn't like about your day? Did you come up against any obstacles today? What were they? *Who* were they? _____
_____
5. Any final thoughts or feelings or things you need to say to complete the day for yourself?
_____
_____
_____
6. Can you let what happened today be the way it was and be the way it was not? (Either a simple "yes" or "no" is okay.) _____

Day Six: _____

Goals for Today

_____
_____
_____

Food Record

_____
_____
_____
_____
_____
_____
_____
_____
_____

Exercise Today

_____
_____
_____
_____
_____
_____
_____
_____

Which "A" list food was added to today's menu?

_____

Which "B" list foods did you not eat?

_____

Protein at each meal?

_____

End-of-the-Day Questions

1. What kind of day did you have? _____
2. What was your energy like? _____
3. Notice any connections between food and mood? Between food and energy? Between food and feelings? _____
4. Any comments about what you liked or didn't like about your day? Did you come up against any obstacles today? What were they? *Who* were they? _____
_____
5. Any final thoughts or feelings or things you need to say to complete the day for yourself?
_____
_____
_____
6. Can you let what happened today be the way it was and be the way it was not? (Either a simple "yes" or "no" is okay.) _____)

Day Seven: _____

Goals for Today

_____
_____
_____

Food Record

_____
_____
_____
_____
_____
_____
_____
_____

Exercise Today

_____
_____
_____
_____
_____
_____
_____

Which "A" list food was added to today's menu?

_____

Which "B" list foods did you not eat?

_____

Protein at each meal?

_____

End-of-the-Day Questions

1. What kind of day did you have? _____
2. What was your energy like? _____
3. Notice any connections between food and mood? Between food and energy? Between food and feelings? _____
4. Any comments about what you liked or didn't like about your day? Did you come up against any obstacles today? What were they? *Who* were they? _____
   _____
5. Any final thoughts or feelings or things you need to say to complete the day for yourself?
   _____
   _____
   _____
6. Can you let what happened today be the way it was and be the way it was not? (Either a simple "yes" or "no" is okay.) _____

Week Five Self-Evaluation Questions

Note: You can write in this section at any time during the week.

What's the one thing you most dislike about your body?

_____

_____

_____

_____

_____

_____

and, more important . . . how would your life be different if—and when—you could change that? How much would you have to change it for your life to be different?

Extra credit question: Would you *really* have to change that body part for your life to be different? Or do you just think you would?

_____

_____

_____

_____

_____

_____

Week Five Round-Up

Note: You can write in this section at any time during the week.

What are you noticing, if anything, from keeping the food journal?

_____

_____

_____

_____

_____

What items came off your to-do list this week?

_____

_____

_____

_____

_____

_____

How are you feeling about doing the program? (Remember, feelings are not facts. You may feel terrific about it, you may hate it. You may feel both! or you may feel anything in between. It's all okay. Just tell the truth about it.)

_____

_____

_____

_____

_____

Anything else you need to say before moving into week six?

_____

_____

_____

_____

_____

_____

_____

_____

_____

_____

_____

_____

_____

WEIGHT AND . . . STRESS

Stress can make you fat.

And there's something you can do about it. It's not something most people think of when they think about weight loss, yet it's free and it's widely available.

It's called sleep and relaxation.

To understand how it works you have to understand a hormone called cortisol.

Cortisol is a hormone that is needed and used by every single cell in the body. It's made by the adrenal glands, two little nut-shaped fellows that sit on top of your kidneys. Among other things, cortisol is an anti-inflammatory (the widely prescribed "cortizone" is a derivative). But cortisol's most famous role is that of a stress hormone.

When your cavemen and cavewomen ancestors saw a wild boar in the woods, their adrenals would shoot a load of cortisol into their bodies, telling them in no uncertain terms that the time had come to pick up a weapon or run like the devil. Cortisol helps the body release sugar into the bloodstream, sugar that can be used for the immediate energy needed for either of the above actions—running or fighting. In fact, during any stressful time—including exercise, by the way—the body releases more cortisol, hence its nickname as a "fight or flight" hormone.

Cortisol is not a "bad" hormone. As with most things, the problem is when it's out of balance. According to Dr. Pamela Peeke, a leading expert in the field, chronic unrelenting stress (of the kind most of us live with everyday) can have a dangerous effect on the body. It makes you more vulnerable to colds, flu, fatigue, and infection, and, if that weren't enough, it gives you a raging appetite in the bargain. Why? Because one of its "purposes" is to help your body "refuel" for the next emergency. Hence, when your body's on constant cortizone overload, you eat. She calls this typical reaction "stress eating," and it has a solid physiological reason: The foods you crave when stressed out (almost always carbohydrates and fat) "replenish the calories used up during the stress response—which, in simplest terms, is one of the main ways that activating the stress response on a constant basis can make you fat."

Now if stress is a factor in weight gain—and it almost certainly is a big one—what's the logical conclusion?

Reduce it! (and with it, your waistline).

Most people are living lives that put an inordinate amount of stress on their systems. We're working too hard. We're managing too many projects (including other people's lives). We're worrying too much. We're sleeping too little. We have too little time for ourselves. Our poor adrenal glands, which were meant to simply be an emergency system for occasional use, have been pressed into overdrive—their owners are running on empty and refueling with junk to keep from noticing. Is it any wonder so many of us are overtired, sleep-deprived, immune-suppressed, depressed, frequently sick, and typically overweight?

So what's the secret weapon? Simple. Stress reduction. (By the way, one of the biggest stressors is continual dieting and worrying about weight!)

Do some deep breathing exercises at least a few times a day. Find something that gives you spiritual solace. Take care of yourself, not just in the obvious ways, but in the ways that only you would understand.

A good place to start is by changing your sleeping habits. Sleep experts estimate that more than half of the U.S. population is walking around in some degree of sleep deprivation. The problem is compounded by our refusal to take time for ourselves—if it's not related to work or family, we just don't do it.

So do it now. Begin by going to bed earlier (staying in bed later is much more difficult for most people). Try banning television from the bedroom. Take a warm bath. Put on soothing music. Eventually, you'll get the hang of it!

Reducing stress is not only good for your health, your immune system, and your psychological well-being, it's good for your waistline as well.

Resources: *Fight Fat After Forty* by Pamela Peeke, M.D.
Tired of Being Tired by Jesse Lynn Hanley, M.D.

Sometimes, even when it seems you are doing everything "right," you are still stuck and nothing seems to be happening. Plateaus are a very natural and normal part of the weight-loss process, frustrating as they may be. Sometimes, though, you just need to be a better detective to find out what's getting in the way of you moving toward your goals. I put this list together not as a "must-do" list, but as a tool for you to use to become a better detective. Not all ten items will apply equally to every person, but giving these strategies a try may indeed produce an "a-ha" experience for you and help you to identify why you've been stuck.

WEEK SIX

Only those willing to go too far will know how far they can go.

—Tom Wolfe

Keep writing. Feelings, impressions, thoughts, poetry, quotes, food, exercise logs, favorite movies, CDs, I don't care. Rename the journal "The Story of Me" if you like.

This is a good time to remind you of the rule that you can't show it to anyone. One of the stumbling blocks some people seem to come up against when they use their journal regularly is curiosity from husbands, wives, lovers, friends and the like. "Hey, watcha got in there?" they ask. "Writing anything about me?" If you tell them it's private, they'll often pout and say some version of the following: "Hey, if you're not writing anything negative in there, how come you won't let me see it?" The answer is simple: You gave your word. It's the rules. Tell them the program only works if you do it that way. Tell them whatever you want. Just know that you can't show it to them. If you even *think*, on some level, that someone else might see it, you will not treat it in the same way.

By the way, it's only "the rules" because you say so. *Your saying so* makes it so. That's probably the most important skill you get to practice in this whole eight-week program. Might as well start with this!

Food Goals: Cutting Back on Sugar

If you haven't already begun to really monitor sugar intake, now's the time to do so. Pay attention to labels. Remember that by law they have to list ingredients by amount, so if you see sugar as the first or second ingredient, that should be a red flag. Manufacturers are sneaky, though. They'll often put several different kinds of sweetener into a product; this way, none of the ingredients by itself is contributing so much to the overall product that "sugar" has to be listed as the first ingredient, but taken together as a whole, that's exactly what's happening. Look for ingredients like "fruit juice concentrate," "high fructose corn syrup," "barley malt," "brown rice syrup," "lactose," "maltodextrin," "maltose," or anything ending in "itol" (mannitol, sorbitol, xylitol). Frightening, isn't it? For some people, cutting down (or cutting out) sugar may just be one of the most profound changes they can make to the diet and may reap the greatest benefits in terms of energy, mood fluctuations, and insulin levels

Exercise Goals

Beginners

- Two days a week: Walking for forty-five minutes a day
- One day a week: Walking for thirty minutes
- Two days a week: Walking for twenty minutes; then crunches, squats, chest presses, one-arm rows, bicep curls, tricep dips, and lateral raises (these are your "weight training days")

Day One	Day Two	Day Three	Day Four	Day Five
Walk 45 min.	Walk 20 min. Crunches Squats Chest presses One-arm rows Bicep curls Tricep dips Lateral raises	Walk 30 min.	Walk 20 min. Crunches Squats Chest presses One-arm rows Bicep curls Tricep dips Lateral raises	Walk 45 min.

Intermediate/Advanced Workout

- Three days a week: Cardio for forty-five minutes (walking, running, stairclimber, or stationary bike)
- Two days a week: Cardio for twenty to thirty minutes (walking, running, stairclimber, or stationary bike); then crunches, squats, chest presses, one-arm rows, bicep curls, tricep dips, and lateral raises, two to three sets each exercise (these are your "weight training days")

- One day a week: Something fun and active such as tennis, tae-bo, golf, group fitness class, yoga, hiking, playing

Day One	Day Two	Day Three	Day Four	Day Five	Day Six
Cardio 45 min.	Cardio 20–30 min.	Cardio 45 min.	Cardio 20–30 min.	Cardio 45 min.	Activity/fun
	Crunches 2–3 sets		Crunches 2–3 sets		
	Squats 2–3 sets		Squats 2–3 sets		
	Chest presses 2–3 sets		Chest presses 2–3 sets		
	One-arm rows 2–3 sets		One-arm rows 2–3 sets		
	Bicep curls 2–3 sets Tricep dips 2–3 sets Lateral raises 2–3 sets		Bicep curls 2–3 sets Tricep dips 2–3 sets Lateral raises 2–3 sets		

OR

- Two days a week: Cardio for forty-five minutes (walking, running, stair-climber, or stationary bike)

PLUS

- Three days: Intermediate Workout "C" (home or gym)
- One day: Something fun and active such as tennis, tae-bo, golf, group fitness class, yoga, hiking, playing

Day One	Day Two	Day Three	Day Four	Day Five	Day Six
Intermediate workout C	Cardio 45 min.	Intermediate workout C	Cardio 45 min.	Intermediate workout C	Activity/fun

To-Do List Goals

Two more things come off this week, but if you want to up the ante, go for it. Hopefully, the to-do list is becoming a regular part of your life by now. It might be a good idea to start looking at some of the bigger things that have been taking up space in your brain, larger projects that you "always wanted to do," and begin to break them up into smaller steps. Then start doing the smaller steps. It's the "to-do" list version of losing weight one pound at a time. When you take actions toward a goal—no matter how small and insignificant the actions may seem—the whole project seems to take on a momentum and energy of its own and stuff starts to happen and fall into place. Sometimes the first actions are as simple as writing down the first steps. Try it.

Day One: _____

Goals for Today

_____
_____
_____

Food Record

_____
_____
_____
_____
_____
_____
_____
_____

Exercise Today

_____
_____
_____
_____
_____
_____
_____
_____

Which "A" list food was added to today's menu?

_____

Which "B" list foods did you not eat?

_____

Protein at each meal?

_____

End-of-the-Day Questions

1. What kind of day did you have? _____
2. What was your energy like? _____
3. Notice any connections between food and mood? Between food and energy? Between food and feelings? _____
4. Any comments about what you liked or didn't like about your day? Did you come up against any obstacles today? What were they? *Who* were they? _____
5. Any final thoughts or feelings or things you need to say to complete the day for yourself?
   _____
   _____
   _____
6. Can you let what happened today be the way it was and be the way it was not? (Either a simple "yes" or "no" is okay.) _____

Day Two: _____

Goals for Today

_____

_____

_____

Food Record

_____

_____

_____

_____

_____

_____

_____

_____

_____

Exercise Today

_____

_____

_____

_____

_____

_____

_____

_____

_____

Which "A" list food was added to today's menu?

_____

Which "B" list foods did you not eat?

_____

Protein at each meal?

_____

End-of-the-Day Questions

1. What kind of day did you have? _____
2. What was your energy like? _____
3. Notice any connections between food and mood? Between food and energy? Between food and feelings? _____
4. Any comments about what you liked or didn't like about your day? Did you come up against any obstacles today? What were they? *Who* were they? _____
   _____
5. Any final thoughts or feelings or things you need to say to complete the day for yourself?
   _____
   _____
   _____
6. Can you let what happened today be the way it was and be the way it was not? (Either a simple "yes" or "no" is okay.) _____

Day Three: _____

Goals for Today

_____

_____

_____

Food Record

_____

_____

_____

_____

_____

_____

_____

_____

Exercise Today

_____

_____

_____

_____

_____

_____

_____

_____

Which "A" list food was added to today's menu?

_____

Which "B" list foods did you not eat?

_____

Protein at each meal?

_____

End-of-the-Day Questions

1. What kind of day did you have? _____

2. What was your energy like? _____

3. Notice any connections between food and mood? Between food and energy? Between food and feelings? _____

4. Any comments about what you liked or didn't like about your day? Did you come up against any obstacles today? What were they? *Who* were they? _____
   _____

5. Any final thoughts or feelings or things you need to say to complete the day for yourself?
   _____
   _____
   _____

6. Can you let what happened today be the way it was and be the way it was not? (Either a simple "yes" or "no" is okay.) _____

Day Four: _____

Goals for Today

_____
_____
_____

Food Record

_____
_____
_____
_____
_____
_____
_____
_____

Exercise Today

_____
_____
_____
_____
_____
_____
_____
_____

Which "A" list food was added to
today's menu?

_____

Which "B" list foods did you not eat?

_____

Protein at each meal?

_____

End-of-the-Day Questions

1. What kind of day did you have? _____
2. What was your energy like? _____
3. Notice any connections between food and mood? Between food and energy? Between food and feelings? _____
4. Any comments about what you liked or didn't like about your day? Did you come up against any obstacles today? What were they? *Who* were they? _____
5. Any final thoughts or feelings or things you need to say to complete the day for yourself?
   _____
   _____
   _____
6. Can you let what happened today be the way it was and be the way it was not? (Either a simple "yes" or "no" is okay.) _____

Day Five: _____

Goals for Today

_____
_____
_____

Food Record

_____
_____
_____
_____
_____
_____
_____
_____
_____

Exercise Today

_____
_____
_____
_____
_____
_____
_____
_____

Which "A" list food was added to today's menu?

_____

Which "B" list foods did you not eat?

_____

Protein at each meal?

_____

End-of-the-Day Questions

1. What kind of day did you have? _____
2. What was your energy like? _____
3. Notice any connections between food and mood? Between food and energy? Between food and feelings? _____
4. Any comments about what you liked or didn't like about your day? Did you come up against any obstacles today? What were they? *Who* were they? _____
5. Any final thoughts or feelings or things you need to say to complete the day for yourself?
   _____
   _____
   _____
6. Can you let what happened today be the way it was and be the way it was not? (Either a simple "yes" or "no" is okay.) _____

Day Six: _____

Goals for Today

_____
_____
_____

Food Record

_____
_____
_____
_____
_____
_____
_____
_____

Exercise Today

_____
_____
_____
_____
_____
_____
_____

Which "A" list food was added to today's menu?

_____

Which "B" list foods did you not eat?

_____

Protein at each meal?

_____

End-of-the-Day Questions

1. What kind of day did you have? _____
2. What was your energy like? _____
3. Notice any connections between food and mood? Between food and energy? Between food and feelings? _____
4. Any comments about what you liked or didn't like about your day? Did you come up against any obstacles today? What were they? *Who* were they? _____
_____
5. Any final thoughts or feelings or things you need to say to complete the day for yourself?
_____
_____
_____
6. Can you let what happened today be the way it was and be the way it was not? (Either a simple "yes" or "no" is okay.) _____

Day Seven: _____

Goals for Today

_____
_____
_____

Food Record

_____
_____
_____
_____
_____
_____
_____

Exercise Today

_____
_____
_____
_____
_____
_____
_____
_____

Which "A" list food was added to today's menu?

_____

Which "B" list foods did you not eat?

_____

Protein at each meal?

_____

End-of-the-Day Questions

1. What kind of day did you have? _____
2. What was your energy like? _____
3. Notice any connections between food and mood? Between food and energy? Between food and feelings? _____
4. Any comments about what you liked or didn't like about your day? Did you come up against any obstacles today? What were they? *Who* were they? _____
_____
5. Any final thoughts or feelings or things you need to say to complete the day for yourself?
_____
_____
_____
6. Can you let what happened today be the way it was and be the way it was not? (Either a simple "yes" or "no" is okay.) _____

Week Six Self-Evaluation Questions

Note: You can write in this section any time during the week.

How much time do you normally take for yourself to take care of *you?* On a daily basis or a weekly basis or as a percentage of your lifetime! Answer any way you choose. Just take a look.

_____

_____

_____

_____

_____

_____

_____

What does "caring for yourself" mean to you? What does it look like?

_____

_____

_____

_____

_____

Week Six Round-Up

Note: You can write in this section any time during the week.

What are you noticing, if anything, from keeping the food journal?

_____

_____

_____

_____

_____

What items came off your to-do list this week?

_____

_____

_____

_____

_____

_____

How are you feeling about doing the program? (Remember, feelings are not facts. You may feel terrific about it, you may hate it. You may feel both! Or you may feel anything in between. It's all okay. Just tell the truth about it.)

_____

_____

_____

_____

_____

_____

Anything else you need to say before moving into week seven?

_____

_____

_____

_____

_____

_____

_____

_____

_____

_____

_____

_____

_____

_____

WEIGHT AND . . . DETOXIFICATION

The liver is the central processing station for virtually everything that comes into the body. It's here that cholesterol is made, fat is broken down and repackaged, and sugar is turned into a storage form called glycogen. Perhaps most important of all, the liver is the body's "detoxification central." All toxins have to go through the liver where they can be neutralized—broken down into less toxic elements and eventually secreted. Toxins that escape this process wind up getting stored in the tissues, and many are stored in fat cells. (One reason why some people don't feel so well in the early stages of fat loss is that their fat has been harboring a lot of these toxic fugitives, and when the fat breaks down, those toxins are released into the bloodstream, like rats deserting a sinking ship.)

The highly processed, highly toxic Western diet makes the situation even worse.

The liver is acting like a tollbooth on a superhighway, and all those toxins are like drivers who don't have an EZ-pass. They jam up the works and slow everything down. This makes it harder for the overworked liver to do its normal jobs of breaking down fat and processing estrogen and other hormones. When detoxification isn't working right, hormone production may be affected. Feeling fatigue is one potential byproduct of this "unhappy liver." Weight gain—or the inability to lose weight—is another.

This is where detoxification diets come in. Many healing modalities recommend this kind of a "spring cleaning" for the liver and digestive system a few times a year, and I think it's a great idea. A detoxification diet is like going to your desk and putting up a temporary sign that says "no more incoming work accepted right now." It's like taking a few days off to really clear out the stuff that's accumulated instead of piling on more. Virtually everyone can benefit from this kind of temporary respite—it's like a vacation for your digestive system.

If this is something that appeals to you there is a lot of material available to help you select a program that works for you. Remember that weight loss is not the purpose of a detoxification diet, but it is often an indirect result because of two reasons: One, by detoxifying you help your digestive and metabolic systems to run more smoothly, and two, because virtually all detoxification plans remove a lot of the foods that give people problems in the first place.

Resources: *The Living Beauty Detox* by Ann Louise Gittleman, M.S., C.N.S.; *The Detox Diet* by Elson Haas, M.D.

WEEK SEVEN

Like a muscle, courage is strengthened by use.
—Ruth Gordon

Life takes guts.
—Lucille Ball

I want you to play the "So, what?" exercise with the facts of your life, and I want you to write down what you find out. Here's how to do it: Take any experience, any feeling, any event, and ask yourself, "What happened?" Don't editorialize, don't judge, don't talk about what *should* have been, don't elaborate. Just say *what happened.* As the detective on the old TV series used to say, "Just the facts ma'am, just the facts." It can be something that happened, or something that is so *right now.* Keep it short and simple. If this is hard to do, *notice* that. Notice how much "story" wants to creep in, even in the simple telling of *what happened,* even when the assignment is *not* to tell a story. (If you're noticing this, you're on your way to a breakthrough.)

When you've finished writing "what happened," or stating "what's so," ask yourself, "So, what?" Write down everything you made that particular "what happened" mean. Be very specific. All the ramifications, everything you think follows from it, everything you think is *inseparable* from it, how you feel about it. Take yourself down the whole, long road you paved for yourself. Follow every nook and cranny. Did "what happened" *cause* your experience, or was it what you *told yourself* about what happened? Start making the distinction.

Now make up a different story. I don't care how hard this is, and for many people it'll be really really hard, do it anyway. A little voice is going to tell you there is *no other story* that could be told out of "what happened." The little voice is lying. Make one up anyway.

Then make up another.

When you're done, make up one more.

Notice anything getting lighter?

If you *didn't* notice it getting lighter, what did you make *that* mean?

Just keep looking. And keep telling the truth about what you're seeing.

When you're done, look some more.

(Psst . . . are you making this mean something very serious?)

Food Goals

It's time to begin to ask yourself some questions about the *quality* of what you're eating. How closely does your food resemble the form in which it would be found in nature? If you're eating meat, how processed is it? Are your eggs from free-ranging chickens? Does the majority of the food you're eating come without a label, or does it have a bar code? Are you eating at least some raw foods each day? Are you beginning to balance how much nutrition and energy is in the food you eat against how convenient it is? Is the balance beginning to shift?

Make your own personal check list of foods that sustain and nourish you. See how many of them you can include on a daily basis.

Make your own personal checklist of foods that take you off-track, that make you feel lousy after you eat them, or that sap your energy and vitality. Maybe they're foods that trigger eating binges, maybe they're foods that give you "brain fog." By now you've probably begun to identify a lot of them. Make your own personal checklist and see how many of them you can eliminate on a daily basis. If you do eat them, make special note of how you feel when you do. And how you feel afterward. Note carefully how you feel when you don't eat them. Notice if you're feeling the same way about those foods as you did when you began the program.

Exercise Goals

Beginners

Now it's time to really up the ante. Two big modifications this week:

- Walking: Go for forty-five minutes three days a week, and thirty minutes on weight training days.
- Weight training: Go through the full circuit* of seven exercises and then *repeat it* for a total of two complete circuits.

*A "circuit" is defined as a complete set of the seven exercises, one set per exercise. Try to move from one exercise to the next with minimum rest in between. When you've completed one set of each of the seven exercises, you've done one circuit.

Crunches (one set)	I
Squats (one set)	I
Chest presses (one set)	I
One-arm rows (one set)	I } = one circuit
Bicep curls (one set)	I
Tricep dips (one set)	I
Lateral raises (one set)	I

Exercise

Beginners

- Two days a week: Walking for forty-five minutes a day
- One day a week: Walking for thirty minutes
- Two days a week: Walking for twenty minutes, then two full "circuits" (these are your "weight training days")
- One day a week: Something fun and active such as tennis, tae-bo, golf, group fitness class, yoga, hiking, playing

Day One	Day Two	Day Three	Day Four	Day Five	Day Six
Walk 45 min.	Walk 20 min. Two full "circuits"	Walk 30 min.	Walk 20 min. Two full "circuits"	Walk 45 min.	Activity/fun

Intermediate/Advanced Workout

- Three days a week: Cardio for forty-five minutes (walking, running, stair-climber, or stationary bike)
- Two days a week: Cardio for twenty to thirty minutes (walking, running, stair-climber, or stationary bike), then three full "circuits" (these are your "weight training" days)

Day One	Day Two	Day Three	Day Four	Day Five
Cardio 45 min.	Cardio 20–30 min. Three full "circuits"	Cardio 45 min.	Cardio 20–30 min. Three full "circuits"	Cardio 45 min.

OR

- Two days a week: Cardio for forty-five minutes (walking, running, stair-climber, or stationary bike)

PLUS

- Three days: Intermediate Workout "C" (home or gym)
- One day: Something fun and active such as tennis, tae-bo, golf, group fitness class, yoga, hiking, playing

Day One	Day Two	Day Three	Day Four	Day Five	Day Six
Intermediate workout C	Cardio 45 min.	Intermediate workout C	Cardio 45 min.	Intermediate workout C	Activity/fun

To-Do List Goals

- This week we're going to do more than just add and remove those items on the list. We're going to look at them a little more closely.
- Pick two things on your to-do list. What stories did you make up about them? What did you make it *mean* if you do them? What did you make it mean if you *didn't* do them? So what?

Do a couple more things on your to-do list. (Or don't.) Notice what you make that mean.

Are you beginning to get the joke?

Keep looking.

Day One: _____

Goals for Today

_____

_____

_____

Food Record

_____

_____

_____

_____

_____

_____

_____

_____

_____

Exercise Today

_____

_____

_____

_____

_____

_____

_____

_____

Are "nourish and sustain" foods on today's menu?

_____

Which "off-track" foods were eliminated?

_____

End-of-the-Day Questions

1. What kind of day did you have? _____
2. What was your energy like? _____
3. Notice any connections between food and mood? Between food and energy? Between food and feelings? _____
4. Any comments about what you liked or didn't like about your day? Did you come up against any obstacles today? What were they? *Who* were they? _____
   _____
5. Any final thoughts or feelings or things you need to say to complete the day for yourself?
   _____
   _____
   _____
6. Can you let what happened today be the way it was and be the way it was not? (Either a simple "yes" or "no" is okay.) _____

Day Two: _____

Goals for Today

_____

_____

_____

Food Record

_____

_____

_____

_____

_____

_____

_____

_____

_____

Exercise Today

_____

_____

_____

_____

_____

_____

_____

_____

_____

Are "nourish and sustain" foods on today's menu?

_____

Which "off-track" foods were eliminated?

_____

End-of-the-Day Questions

1. What kind of day did you have? _____
2. What was your energy like? _____
3. Notice any connections between food and mood? Between food and energy? Between food and feelings? _____
4. Any comments about what you liked or didn't like about your day? Did you come up against any obstacles today? What were they? *Who* were they? _____
_____
5. Any final thoughts or feelings or things you need to say to complete the day for yourself?
_____
_____
_____
6. Can you let what happened today be the way it was and be the way it was not? (Either a simple "yes" or "no" is okay.) _____

Day Three: _____

Goals for Today

_____

_____

_____

Food Record

_____

_____

_____

_____

_____

_____

_____

_____

_____

_____

Exercise Today

_____

_____

_____

_____

_____

_____

_____

_____

Are "nourish and sustain" foods on today's menu?

_____

Which "off-track" foods were eliminated?

_____

End-of-the-Day Questions

1. What kind of day did you have? _____
2. What was your energy like? _____
3. Notice any connections between food and mood? Between food and energy? Between food and feelings? _____
4. Any comments about what you liked or didn't like about your day? Did you come up against any obstacles today? What were they? *Who* were they? _____
_____
5. Any final thoughts or feelings or things you need to say to complete the day for yourself?
_____
_____
_____
6. Can you let what happened today be the way it was and be the way it was not? (Either a simple "yes" or "no" is okay.) _____

Day Four: _____

Goals for Today

_____
_____
_____

Food Record

_____
_____
_____
_____
_____
_____
_____
_____
_____
_____

Exercise Today

_____
_____
_____
_____
_____
_____
_____
_____

Are "nourish and sustain" foods on today's menu?

_____

Which "off-track" foods were eliminated?

_____

End-of-the-Day Questions

1. What kind of day did you have? _____
2. What was your energy like? _____
3. Notice any connections between food and mood? Between food and energy? Between food and feelings? _____
4. Any comments about what you liked or didn't like about your day? Did you come up against any obstacles today? What were they? *Who* were they? _____
5. Any final thoughts or feelings or things you need to say to complete the day for yourself?
   _____
   _____
   _____
6. Can you let what happened today be the way it was and be the way it was not? (Either a simple "yes" or "no" is okay.) _____

Day Five: _____

Goals for Today

_____
_____
_____

Food Record

_____
_____
_____
_____
_____
_____
_____
_____

Exercise Today

_____
_____
_____
_____
_____
_____
_____
_____

Are "nourish and sustain" foods on today's menu?

_____

Which "off-track" foods were eliminated?

_____

End-of-the-Day Questions

1. What kind of day did you have? _____
2. What was your energy like? _____
3. Notice any connections between food and mood? Between food and energy? Between food and feelings? _____
4. Any comments about what you liked or didn't like about your day? Did you come up against any obstacles today? What were they? *Who* were they? _____
_____
5. Any final thoughts or feelings or things you need to say to complete the day for yourself?
_____
_____
_____
6. Can you let what happened today be the way it was and be the way it was not? (Either a simple "yes" or "no" is okay.) _____

Day Six: _____

Goals for Today

_____
_____
_____

Food Record

_____
_____
_____
_____
_____
_____
_____
_____
_____

Exercise Today

_____
_____
_____
_____
_____
_____
_____
_____
_____

Are "nourish and sustain" foods on today's menu?

_____

Which "off-track" foods were eliminated?

_____

End-of-the-Day Questions

1. What kind of day did you have? _____
2. What was your energy like? _____
3. Notice any connections between food and mood? Between food and energy? Between food and feelings? _____
4. Any comments about what you liked or didn't like about your day? Did you come up against any obstacles today? What were they? *Who* were they? _____
_____
5. Any final thoughts or feelings or things you need to say to complete the day for yourself?
_____
_____
_____
6. Can you let what happened today be the way it was and be the way it was not? (Either a simple "yes" or "no" is okay.) _____

Day Seven: _____

Goals for Today

_____

_____

_____

Food Record

_____

_____

_____

_____

_____

_____

_____

_____

_____

Exercise Today

_____

_____

_____

_____

_____

_____

_____

_____

Are "nourish and sustain" foods on today's menu?

_____

Which "off-track" foods were eliminated?

_____

End-of-the-Day Questions

1. What kind of day did you have? _____
2. What was your energy like? _____
3. Notice any connections between food and mood? Between food and energy? Between food and feelings? _____
4. Any comments about what you liked or didn't like about your day? Did you come up against any obstacles today? What were they? *Who* were they? _____
_____
5. Any final thoughts or feelings or things you need to say to complete the day for yourself?
_____
_____
_____
6. Can you let what happened today be the way it was and be the way it was not? (Either a simple "yes" or "no" is okay.) _____)

Week Seven Self-Evaluation Questions

Note: You can write in this section at any time during the week.

What does your weight "say" about you?

_____

_____

_____

_____

_____

_____

_____

Do *you* say that or does your weight? Who made that up? (Helpful hint: If you think "someone else" or "society" made it up, how much do you agree with it? Who made *that* story up?)

_____

_____

_____

_____

_____

_____

Week Seven Round-Up

Note: You can write in this section at any time during the week.

What are you noticing, if anything, from keeping the food journal?

_____

_____

_____

_____

_____

What items came off your to-do list this week? And what did you notice about what you made that mean?

_____

_____

_____

_____

_____

_____

_____

How are you feeling about doing the program? (Remember, feelings are not facts. You may feel terrific about it, you may hate it. You may feel both! Or you may feel anything in between. It's all okay. Just tell the truth about it.)

_____

_____

_____

_____

_____

_____

_____

Anything else you need to say before moving into week eight?

_____

_____

_____

_____

_____

_____

_____

_____

_____

WEEK EIGHT

Perfectionism is self-abuse of the highest order.

—ANNE WILSON SCHAEF

Think of someone you know in your life who is a "procrastinator." Maybe it's you, or at least maybe it was you before you began this book. Now write down what being a procrastinator *means*. What do you know about a person who is a procrastinator? What's true about him? Take a minute and jot down what comes to mind before reading further.

Good. Did you say that that person who procrastinates are lazy? Unmotivated? Fearful of success? Irresponsible? Come on, fess up.

Now I'm going to tell you something. Procrastinators are wise. They take time to evaluate. They are thinkers and seekers. They're romantic dreamers. They take longer to get stuff done, but so what? They're also more likely to come up with far more creative stuff than the average person when they finally do get around to taking action.

Now I'm going to tell you one more thing. *I just made that up.* Just like *you* made up that the procrastinator is lazy and unmotivated. Neither story is any more "true" than the other.

And you know what else? Being a procrastinator—or being fat or being tall or being beautiful or having one leg or winning the French Open or breaking up with a lover— doesn't mean anything except what *you say it means*.

Beginning to get the point?

Food Goals

It's been my experience that people are in very different places with their food plans by the time we get to the eighth week. Remember that our goal is to discover what works and tell the truth about it. For most people, what works is going to be some combination of high-quality protein, traditional and nourishing fats, vegetables, and fruits, and perhaps limited amounts of low-sugar, high-fiber starches like oatmeal and sweet potatoes and beans. The exact amounts and proportions are going to ultimately have to be your own design, but by now you have everything you need to craft a food plan that honors the unique needs of your body. Remember once again that losing weight is a process, not an event.

When something gets in the way, look it in the eye, tell the truth about it, disarm it, and move on.

As Winston Churchill said, in his address to the graduating class of Oxford University, "*Never, never, ever give up.*"

Exercise Goals

Beginners

- Three days a week: Walking for forty-five minutes
- Two days a week: Walking for thirty to forty-five minutes, then two full "circuits" (these are your "weight training days")
- One day a week: Something fun and active such as tennis, tae-bo, group fitness class, golf, yoga, hiking, playing

Day One	Day Two	Day Three	Day Four	Day Five	Day Six
Walk 45 min.	Walk 30–45 min. Two full "circuits	Walk 45 min.	Walk 30–45 min. Two full "circuits"	Walk 45 min.	Activity/fun

Intermediate/Advanced Workout

- Three days a week: Cardio for forty-five minutes (walking, running, stairclimber, or stationary bike)
- Two days a week: Cardio for thirty to forty-five minutes (walking, running, stairclimber, or stationary bike), then three full "circuits" (these are your "weight training days")

- One day: Something fun and active such as tennis, tae-bo, golf, group fitness class, yoga, hiking, playing

Day One	Day Two	Day Three	Day Four	Day Five	Day Six
Cardio 45 min.	Cardio 30–45 min.	Cardio 45 min.	Cardio 30–45 min.	Cardio 45 min.	Activity/fun
	Three full "circuits"		Three full "circuits"		

OR

- Two days a week: Cardio for forty-five minutes (walking, running, stair-climber, or stationary bike)

PLUS

- Three days: Intermediate Workout "C" (home or gym)
- One day: Something fun and active such as tennis, tae-bo, golf, group fitness class, yoga, hiking, playing

Day One	Day Two	Day Three	Day Four	Day Five	Day Six
Intermediate workout C	Cardio 45 min.	Intermediate workout C	Cardio 45 min.	Intermediate workout C	Activity/fun

To-Do List Goals

Make up an assignment for the To-Do List. Give your word that you're going to do that assignment. I suggest saying it out loud. The assignment can be that you're going to do X number of things on the list, or it can be that you *won't* do X number of things on the list. Doesn't matter. All that matters is one thing: You *say* it, you *do* it. Period.

Look, your commitment to keep your word only matters because *you say it does*. The universe *does not care* whether you keep your word or not. It will go on anyway, just as gravity will keep on being gravity whether you agree with it or not. Your word only matters because you—and perhaps the people around you—have agreed to *make* it matter. Whether or not you want to *keep* that agreement is up to you. I'm hoping that over the last eight weeks you will have begun to notice that you have a lot more power—and things work out a lot better—when you keep your agreements.

That's what the whole to-do list experience has been about.

Day One: _____

Goals for Today

_____
_____
_____

Food Record

_____
_____
_____
_____
_____
_____
_____
_____
_____

Exercise Today

_____
_____
_____
_____
_____
_____
_____
_____

Are "nourish and sustain" foods on today's menu?

_____

Which "off-track" foods were eliminated?

_____

End-of-the-Day Questions

1. What kind of day did you have? _____
2. What was your energy like? _____
3. Notice any connections between food and mood? Between food and energy? Between food and feelings? _____
4. Any comments about what you liked or didn't like about your day? Did you come up against any obstacles today? What were they? *Who* were they? _____
5. Any final thoughts or feelings or things you need to say to complete the day for yourself?
_____
_____
_____
6. Can you let what happened today be the way it was and be the way it was not? (Either a simple "yes" or "no" is okay.) _____

Day Two: _____

Goals for Today

_____

_____

_____

Food Record

_____

_____

_____

_____

_____

_____

_____

_____

Exercise Today

_____

_____

_____

_____

_____

_____

_____

_____

Are "nourish and sustain" foods on today's menu?

_____

Which "off-track" foods were eliminated?

_____

End-of-the-Day Questions

1. What kind of day did you have? _____
2. What was your energy like? _____
3. Notice any connections between food and mood? Between food and energy? Between food and feelings? _____
4. Any comments about what you liked or didn't like about your day? Did you come up against any obstacles today? What were they? *Who* were they? _____
   _____
5. Any final thoughts or feelings or things you need to say to complete the day for yourself?
   _____
   _____
   _____
6. Can you let what happened today be the way it was and be the way it was not? (Either a simple "yes" or "no" is okay.) _____

Day Three: _____

Goals for Today

_____

_____

_____

Food Record

_____

_____

_____

_____

_____

_____

_____

_____

_____

Exercise Today

_____

_____

_____

_____

_____

_____

_____

_____

Are "nourish and sustain" foods on today's menu?

_____

Which "off-track" foods were eliminated?

_____

End-of-the-Day Questions

1. What kind of day did you have? _____

2. What was your energy like? _____

3. Notice any connections between food and mood? Between food and energy? Between food and feelings? _____

4. Any comments about what you liked or didn't like about your day? Did you come up against any obstacles today? What were they? *Who* were they? _____
   _____

5. Any final thoughts or feelings or things you need to say to complete the day for yourself?
   _____
   _____
   _____

6. Can you let what happened today be the way it was and be the way it was not? (Either a simple "yes" or "no" is okay.) _____

Day Four: _____

Goals for Today

_____

_____

_____

Food Record

_____

_____

_____

_____

_____

_____

_____

_____

Exercise Today

_____

_____

_____

_____

_____

_____

_____

_____

Are "nourish and sustain" foods on today's menu?

_____

Which "off-track" foods were eliminated?

_____

End-of-the-Day Questions

1. What kind of day did you have? _____

2. What was your energy like? _____

3. Notice any connections between food and mood? Between food and energy? Between food and feelings? _____

4. Any comments about what you liked or didn't like about your day? Did you come up against any obstacles today? What were they? *Who* were they? _____

5. Any final thoughts or feelings or things you need to say to complete the day for yourself?

_____

_____

_____

6. Can you let what happened today be the way it was and be the way it was not? (Either a simple "yes" or "no" is okay.) _____

Day Five: _____

Goals for Today

_____

_____

_____

Food Record

_____

_____

_____

_____

_____

_____

_____

_____

Exercise Today

_____

_____

_____

_____

_____

_____

_____

_____

Are "nourish and sustain" foods on today's menu?

_____

Which "off-track" foods were eliminated?

_____

End-of-the-Day Questions

1. What kind of day did you have? _____

2. What was your energy like? _____

3. Notice any connections between food and mood? Between food and energy? Between food and feelings? _____

4. Any comments about what you liked or didn't like about your day? Did you come up against any obstacles today? What were they? *Who* were they? _____

   _____

5. Any final thoughts or feelings or things you need to say to complete the day for yourself?

   _____

   _____

   _____

6. Can you let what happened today be the way it was and be the way it was not? (Either a simple "yes" or "no" is okay.) _____

Day Six: _____

Goals for Today

_____
_____
_____

Food Record

_____
_____
_____
_____
_____
_____
_____
_____
_____

Exercise Today

_____
_____
_____
_____
_____
_____
_____
_____

Are "nourish and sustain" foods on today's menu?

_____

Which "off-track" foods were eliminated?

_____

End-of-the-Day Questions

1. What kind of day did you have? _____
2. What was your energy like? _____
3. Notice any connections between food and mood? Between food and energy? Between food and feelings? _____
4. Any comments about what you liked or didn't like about your day? Did you come up against any obstacles today? What were they? *Who* were they? _____
   _____
5. Any final thoughts or feelings or things you need to say to complete the day for yourself?
   _____
   _____
   _____
6. Can you let what happened today be the way it was and be the way it was not? (Either a simple "yes" or "no" is okay.) _____

Day Seven: _____

Goals for Today

_____
_____
_____

Food Record

_____
_____
_____
_____
_____
_____
_____
_____
_____

Exercise Today

_____
_____
_____
_____
_____
_____
_____
_____

Are "nourish and sustain" foods on today's menu?

_____

Which "off-track" foods were eliminated?

_____

End-of-the-Day Questions

1. What kind of day did you have? _____

2. What was your energy like? _____

3. Notice any connections between food and mood? Between food and energy? Between food and feelings? _____

4. Any comments about what you liked or didn't like about your day? Did you come up against any obstacles today? What were they? *Who* were they? _____
_____

5. Any final thoughts or feelings or things you need to say to complete the day for yourself?
_____
_____
_____

6. Can you let what happened today be the way it was and be the way it was not? (Either a simple "yes" or "no" is okay.) _____

Week Eight: Self-Evaluation Questions

Note: You can write in this section any time during the week

What would you most like to be remembered for?

_____

_____

_____

_____

_____

_____

What would you most like people to say about you?

_____

_____

_____

_____

_____

What are you doing to make that happen?

_____

_____

_____

_____

_____

_____

_____

_____

_____

Week Eight Round-Up

Note: You can write in this section at any time during the week.

What have you noticed, if anything, from keeping the food journal for the past eight weeks?

_____
_____
_____
_____
_____
_____
_____

Any comments about the to-do list this week?

_____
_____
_____
_____
_____
_____
_____

Is there anything else you need to say before finishing the eighth week?

_____
_____
_____
_____
_____
_____
_____
_____

Graduations are commencements, not endings.

—Dr. Bernie Siegal

You are a child of God.

Your playing small does not serve the world.

There is nothing enlightened about shrinking so that other people won't feel insecure around you.

We were born to make manifest the glory of God that is within us

It is not just in some of us; it is in everyone.

And as we let our own light shine, we unconsciously give other people permission to do the same.

As we are liberated from our own fear, our presence automatically liberates others.

—Nelson Mandela

If God came out of heaven and told you that what you are doing in your life right now is exactly what He wanted you to do and that where you are right now is exactly where He wanted you to be, you would be happy.

Be happy.

—Werner Erhard

Welcome to your life.

It is your finest creation.

There is no one else on earth who could have created it.

You are exactly where you are supposed to be.

What is, is.

What ain't, ain't.

Let the games begin.

— JONNY

WORKOUT NOTES

WORKOUT NOTES

WORKOUT NOTES

WORKOUT NOTES

WORKOUT NOTES